£42.00
4/86
14.00
26/X
TELEPEN
81 8810126 8
DILEWYD O STOC
WITHDRAWN FROM STOCK
CPC UCW
LLYFRGELL
LIBRARY
ABERYSTWYTH
AF751566

Current Topics in Research on Synapses

Volume 3

Editorial Board

M.J. Berry
Department of Anatomy
Guys Hospital Medical School
London Bridge
London SE1 9KT, UK

H.F. Bradford
Department of Biochemistry
Imperial College
London SW7 2AZ, UK

E.M. Burns
College of Nursing
University of Iowa
Iowa City, Iowa 52242, USA

C.W. Cotman
Department of Psychobiology
University of California
Irvine, California 92717, USA

D.R. Curtis
Department of Pharmacology
John Curtin School of Medical Research
Australian National University
Canberra City, A.C.T. 2601, Australia

W.T. Greenough
Department of Psychology
University of Illinois at Urbana-Champaign
603 East Daniel
Champaign, Illinois 61820, USA

G.D. Pappas
Department of Anatomy
University of Illinois at the Medical Center
808 South Wood Street
Chicago, Illinois 60612, USA

Current Topics in Research on Synapses

Volume 3

Editor

D. Gareth Jones

Department of Anatomy
University of Otago
Dunedin, New Zealand

Alan R. Liss, Inc., New York

Address all Inquiries to the Publisher
Alan R. Liss, Inc., 41 East 11th Street, New York, NY 10003

Copyright © 1986 Alan R. Liss, Inc.

Printed in the United States of America.

Under the conditions stated below the owner of copyright for this book hereby grants permission to users to make photocopy reproductions of any part or all of its contents for personal or internal organizational use, or for personal or internal use of specific clients. This consent is given on the condition that the copier pay the stated per-copy fee through the Copyright Clearance Center, Incorporated, 27 Congress Street, Salem, MA 01970, as listed in the most current issue of "Permissions to Photocopy" (Publisher's Fee List, distributed by CCC, Inc.), for copying beyond that permitted by sections 107 or 108 of the US Copyright Law. This consent does not extend to other kinds of copying, such as copying for general distribution, for advertising or promotional purposes, for creating new collective works, or for resale.
Library of Congress Cataloging in Publication Data
Main entry under title.

ISBN 0-8451-3902-9 • ISSN 0747-5454

Coleg Prifysgol Cymru
The University College Of Wales
Aberystwyth
Acc. No. 8188101268
Class No. QP 364 C9

Contents

4 Structural Plasticity of Synaptic Contacts in the Central Nervous System

Contributors

David K. Bilkey
Department of Psychology and The Neuroscience Centre, University of Otago, Dunedin, New Zealand **[1]**

Elizabeth M. Burns
College of Nursing, The University of Iowa, Iowa City, Iowa 52242, USA **[29]**

Graham V. Goddard
Department of Psychology and The Neuroscience Centre, University of Otago, Dunedin, New Zealand **[1]**

F.H. Güldner
Department of Anatomy, Monash University, Clayton, Victoria 3168, Australia **[147]**

Kristy Kultas-Ilinsky
Department of Anatomy, The University of Iowa College of Medicine, Iowa City, Iowa 52242, USA **[77]**

Igor A. Ilinsky
Department of Anatomy, The University of Iowa College of Medicine, Iowa City, Iowa 52242, USA **[77]**

S.C. Phillips
Department of Anatomy, Monash University, Clayton, Victoria 3168, Australia **[147]**

The number in brackets designates the first page number of the contributor's chapter.

Contents of Volume 1

Contents of Volume 2

Preface

The chapters of this volume reflect both the diversity of interests and disciplines of those involved in synaptic studies, and also the relevance of many of these studies to human concerns. For instance, Bilkey and Goddard concentrate on long-term potentiation (LTP), a candidate as one of the synaptic changes responsible for memory. They review LTP in terms of functional and morphological considerations, and ask whether present concepts are adequate to account for the phenomenon. Their review, therefore, is a call for further exploration and for a refinement of current concepts.

In considering the effects of ethanol on synaptic membrane biochemistry, Burns places the scientific data within the social context of the fetal alcohol syndrome (FAS). This leads her to a discussion of the heightened susceptibility of rapidly developing synaptic structures during the brain growth spurt, and to a consideration of various developmental issues including the existence of vulnerable periods during brain ontogeny, and the properties of developing pre- and postsynaptic membranes. She then looks in detail at the potentially damaging effects of ethanol on membrane structure and function, and at the relevance of animal models for these investigations.

Although Güldner and Phillips confine their attention to synaptic morphology, the significance of their discussion stems from the plasticity demonstrated by synaptic appositions. This, in turn, is relevant to the much broader question of neural plasticity. Güldner and Phillips discuss the evidence available regarding the plasticity demonstrated by presynaptic dense projections, the synaptic appositions (in terms of their length and curvature), and the postsynaptic densities. In particular, they put forward the hypothesis that the amount of postsynaptic density material is proportional to the efficiency of excitatory synapses.

The chapter by Kultas-Ilinsky and Ilinsky summarizes the data available on the organization of the motor thalamic nuclei in different species. Their treatment of this topic is characterized by a desire to understand the complexity of synaptic arrangements, and to describe changes that may have occurred in the course of evolutionary specialization. Here again then, the authors have attempted to place their specific interests in a broader perspective—in this case a comparative one.

D. Gareth Jones

1

Long-Term Potentiation as a Synaptic Event

David K. Bilkey and Graham V. Goddard

Long-term potentiation (LTP) is a synaptic change induced by short-duration, high-frequency afferent activity. It is most commonly studied in the hippocampus, where the defining changes in field potentials may last for periods of several weeks or more. In this chapter we describe two main aspects of LTP: an increase in the synaptic depolarization of dendrites and an additional increase in the cellular responses to this depolarization. The spatial and temporal characteristics of LTP-inducing stimuli are discussed in terms of whether afferent activity with similar characteristics can occur in the behaving animal. We review the various studies that have been made of the morphological correlates of LTP and conclude that the magnitude of the changes observed are probably too small to account for the large changes in EPSP seen after LTP induction. They may, however, relate to the other, cellular components of LTP.

From the Department of Psychology and The Neuroscience Centre, University of Otago, Dunedin, New Zealand.

Current Topics in Research on Synapses, Volume 3, pages 1–27 **© 1986 Alan R. Liss, Inc.**

U.C.W. ABERYSTWYTH LIBRARY

1 INTRODUCTION

Since the time of Tanzi (1893), cited Cajal [1], a leading candidate for the reductionist account of memory has been an increase in the efficacy of synaptic transmission. The theory, even in its most general terms, asserts that the synaptic changes responsible for memory occur in the relevant regions of the brain, are activated by physiological events, and are long-lasting. At the present time, no known phenomena have been shown to meet all these requirements, but one, known variously as long-term potentiation, long-lasting potentiation, enhancement, and long-term enhancement, appears to be a likely candidate [2,3]. This phenomenon has attracted much attention in recent years, and in this chapter we shall review its physiological properties and comment on the attempts to find its morphological substrate. We shall use the term long-term potentiation (LTP) as this seems to be the one most commonly used.

2 PHYSIOLOGICAL PARAMETERS

2.1 Nature of LTP

LTP is most readily induced and observed in the hippocampus [4], an area of the brain with apparent involvement in the processes of learning and memory [5], which, because of its laminar cytoarchitecture [6], sustains large field potentials that are readily recorded. The latter feature is an important consideration in LTP research, as the difficulties encountered with attempts to monitor intracellular activity for long time periods do not apply in extracellular recording of field potentials, and yet the subcellular components of the events can be inferred when the field potentials are generated in redundantly connected, laminated cytoarchitecture.

In particular, the synapses of the perforant path-dentate gyrus of the rat hippocampus support high levels of LTP and have received extensive investigation. In this preparation, a stimulating electrode is located among the perforant path afferents to the dentate gyrus, usually at the level of the angular bundle, and an extracellular recording electrode is located in the dentate hilus (Fig. 1). Single-pulse stimulation evokes characteristic field potentials (Fig. 2), in which the early, positive-going component reflects the depolarization of the granule cell dendrites, referred to as the field excitatory postsynaptic potential (EPSP), and at sufficiently high stimulus intensities a slightly later and superimposed negative-going component reflects the synchronous activation of a number of granule cells [7] and is referred to as the population spike.

The slope of the rising portion of the EPSP can be used as an approximate measure of the current flowing into the cells in the synaptic region of the molecular layer, and out of the cells, primarily in the granular layer; the height of the population spike reflects the number of cells activated by this averaged synaptic drive. As long as the recording elec-

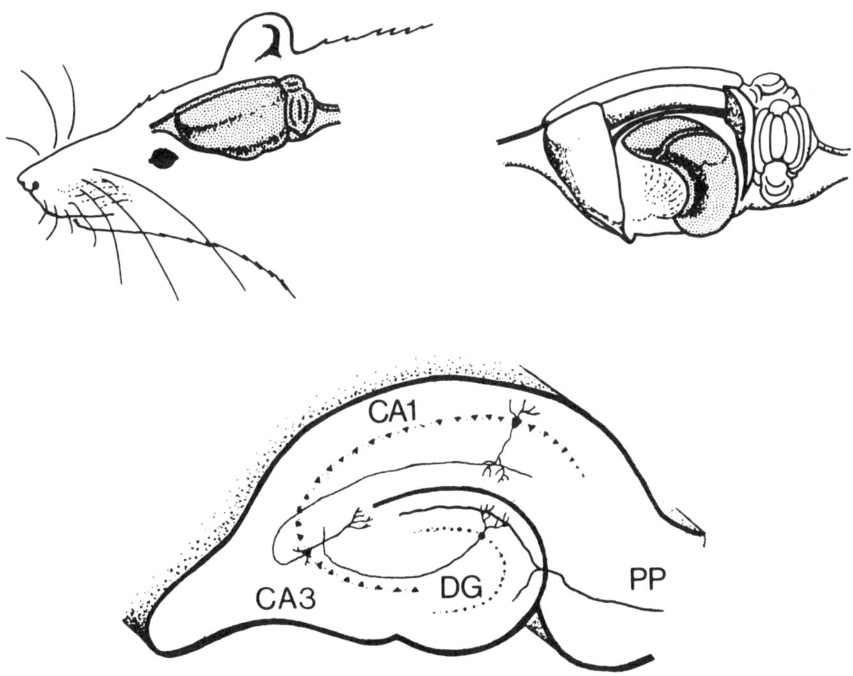

Fig. 1. View of the rat brain dissected to show the location of the left hippocampus (top). A section through the hippocampus (bottom) shows the perforant path (PP) fibers innervating the granule cells of the dentate gyrus (DG). The pyramidal cells of area CA3 and CA1 are also shown.

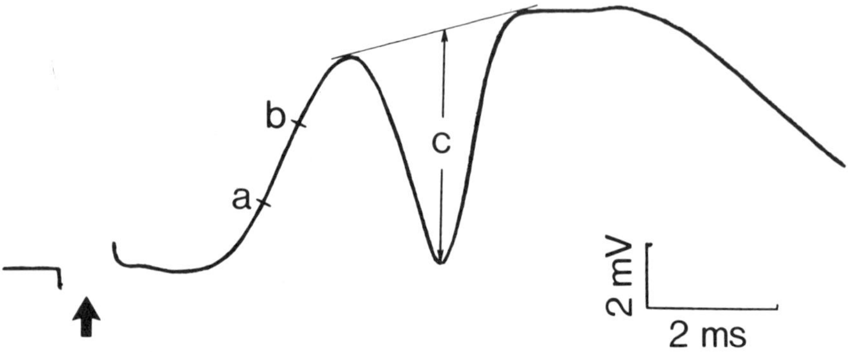

Fig. 2. The characteristic field potential recorded in the hilus of the dentate gyrus after a test pulse (arrow) is applied to the medial perforant path. The amplitude of the field EPSP is inferred from the slope of the rising portion of the waveform between points a and b. The height of the population spike is measured at c.

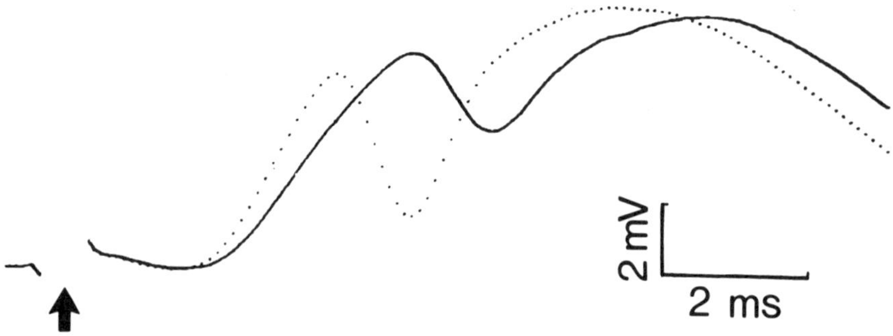

Fig. 3. Waveforms recorded after the application of a fixed intensity test pulse (arrow) before (solid line) and 20 min after (dotted line) the induction of LTP. Note the increase in EPSP slope, the increase in population spike height, and the decrease in population spike latency following induction of LTP.

trode does not move more than a few microns, test pulses of constant intensity will evoke field potentials that remain constant in these measures over long periods of time.

Application of a short burst of high-frequency stimulation, for example 10 pulses at 400 Hz, will result in a lasting increase in the field potentials evoked by the constant-intensity test pulses (Fig. 3). The slope of the rising phase of the EPSP is greater, indicating an increase in synaptic drive, and the population spike height is larger, indicating an increase in the number of cells activated by this drive. A decrease in the population

[16]. They hypothesize that hindbrain structures may utilize a different form of memory mechanism from forebrain areas. Better descriptions of the nature of the "lower nervous system LTP" phenomenon will be needed to test the viability of this hypothesis.

2.3 LTP Induction

Unfortunately, at the present time a complete study of the stimulus parameters required for LTP induction in the hippocampus, where it is best studied, has yet to be undertaken. The interaction of such factors as frequency, train duration, and stimulus intensity have not been explored fully. There have, however, been several studies that have catalogued the broad range of stimulation parameters needed to induce the effect. Dunwiddie and Lynch compared the ability of trains of 100 pulses, delivered at frequencies of 1–100 Hz, to induce LTP in the CA1 region of the hippocampal slice preparation [13]. They found that 100-Hz trains were most effective at producing LTP, lower frequencies were proportionally less effective, and the lowest frequency tested, 1 Hz, produced depression instead of LTP. Although disagreement exists about the effect of trains of 1 Hz and below [33], similar findings for the middle and higher frequencies were obtained in a study by Barrionuevo et al. [34] and Douglas and Goddard [8] in anesthetized rats.

The long-lasting effect known as kindling [35], which eventually results in generalized seizures, can also be induced by stimulation at these frequencies. Although LTP may be an important factor in the generation of kindling [36,37], LTP can be obtained in the absence of kindling and is independent of seizure activity.

Douglas has demonstrated that a frequency of 400–500 Hz appears to be optimal for inducing LTP in the perforant path–granule cell synapses [38]. When stimulation was applied at frequencies of greater than 500 Hz, a comparatively greater number of pulses was required in the train before LTP was induced. This frequency asymptote corresponds with the frequency above which the axons are unlikely to generate an action potential for each pulse within the train. The effects of long stimulation trains on LTP induction have not been fully explored, but at the lower limits it has been determined that LTP can be induced by stimulation that mimics physiological levels of discharge, for example, 3–7 pulses at 400 Hz [38]. Discharge rates within this LTP-inducing range have been described for neurons in many parts of the nervous system including the entorhinal cortex. Unfortunately, the available studies of the discharge rates of entorhinal cells [39] have not demonstrated that the cells recorded were also those giving rise to the perforant path fibers.

2.4 Cooperativity

We have described how LTP induction occurs only if the afferent input is within certain temporal limits, as met by the requirement of high-frequency stimulation. It is also apparent that LTP induction requires the input to conform to certain spatial limits as well. Spatial interactions are important in many memory models. For example, Hebb's theory of cell assemblies proposes that a strengthening of synaptic potency occurs when an afferent fiber cooperates in the activation of a postsynaptic cell [40]. In such a case, the afferent fiber is an associate of other afferents that are coactive in bringing the postsynaptic cell above its discharge threshold. A mechanism such as this, it is thought, could account for many forms of associative learning.

LTP appears to require a slightly different form of associative interaction. When high-frequency stimulation is applied to the perforant path, a minimum stimulus intensity is required before LTP of perforant path-granule cell synapses occurs. This LTP threshold is considerably above that required to produce a synaptic response in the dentate gyrus [41]. As stimulus intensity is increased, more afferent fibers are activated, and thus it appears that a certain minimum number of converging inputs must be coactive at a high frequency before LTP occurs. This requirement has been called cooperativity [41]. The cooperativity effect can also be demonstrated between two separate afferent pathways. Concurrent, but spatially separate, high-frequency stimulation of the converging medial and lateral subcomponents of the perforant path produces LTP when the stimulus intensities are set at too weak a level to produce LTP when either path is stimulated alone (Fig. 4). Similar forms of cooperativity have been demonstrated in several other hippocampal pathways, for example in the dentate gyrus molecular layer of the slice preparation [42], in the ipsilateral and crossed components of the perforant path [43,44], and in the CA1 region [45]. The temporal relationship required between the activity in the two pathways is very strict and cooperativity does not occur unless the stimulus trains either overlap or occur within a few milliseconds of each other [44,46].

Two recent studies report some form of associative interaction between the perforant path and septohippocampal afferents to the dentate gyrus [47,48]. Such a finding is of interest, as it suggests that cooperativity can occur between afferents of different anatomical and neurochemical makeup. However, not all laboratories have agreed on the nature of this effect and it may be a different class of phenomenon from the perforant path and the CA1 cooperativity effects. For example, it may involve a

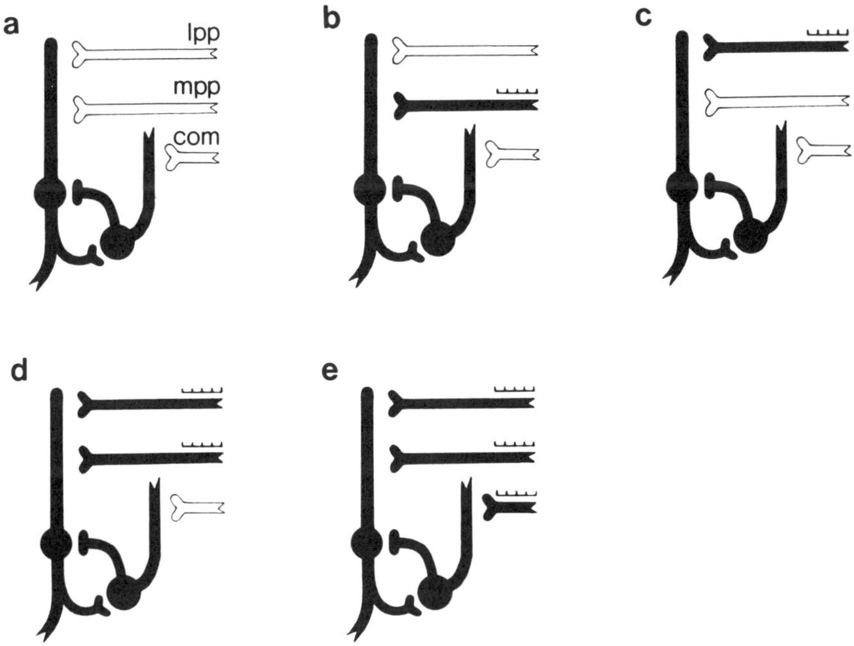

Fig. 4. Schematic diagram illustrating afferents to a dentate gyrus granule cell and to the inhibitory interneuron mediating its recurrent inhibition, and showing how cooperative effects are demonstrated in this preparation. a. The lateral perforant path (lpp) projects to the outer third of the granule cell dendrites, and the medial perforant path (mpp) projects to the middle third. Commissural fibers (com) from the contralateral hilus project to the interneuron dendrites. Weak high-frequency stimulation of the mpp (b) or the lpp (c) alone will not induce LTP, whereas the same stimuli applied concurrently to both pathways (d) will induce LTP. If the commissural input is also stimulated concurrently (e), LTP does not occur.

separate medial septal-entorhinal cortex pathway [49] or result from septal effects on hilar interneurons [50].

McNaughton et al. [51] have calculated that approximately 400 fibers must be coactive in order to produce a granule cell action potential. Since the population spike threshold is also very close to the LTP-induction threshold [41], we assume that a similar number of fibers must be coactive at high frequency in order to produce LTP. Braitenberg and Schuz have estimated that each granule cell receives as many as 18,000 synapses [52]. Therefore, it would appear that a minimum proportion of approximately 2.2% of the synapses on any target granule cell must be coactive briefly at high frequency before LTP occurs.

The close relationship between action potential threshold and LTP threshold suggests that postsynaptic cell activation may be required for LTP induction, in much the same way as in the Hebb's proposal [40] that synaptic connections are strengthened when active at the time of the postsynaptic action potential. Some support for this proposal is implicit in the finding that high-frequency stimulation of the contralateral hilus, combined with high-frequency perforant path stimulation, will block LTP of the perforant path–granule cell synapses [53]. Fibers from the contralateral hilus appear to activate the inhibitory interneurons mediating feed-forward and recurrent inhibition of the dentate gyrus granule cells. Stimulation of the contralateral hilus, therefore, leads to inhibition of the granule cells [54]. Whether this finding confirms the Hebb hypothesis requiring postsynaptic cell action potentials remains equivocal, as the precise mechanism of this blocking is unclear, and other experiments manipulating the action potentials have failed to support this interpretation [53,55] (but see Scharfman and Sarvey [56]). Whatever the case, however, it is of interest that LTP can be prevented by a type of negative cooperativity from an inhibitory pathway.

2.5 Duration of LTP

Several studies report LTP lasting for very long periods of time after the high-frequency stimulation that induced it. Bliss and Gardner-Medwin [2] report examples of LTP in the perforant path–granule cell synapses of the rabbit lasting for 1–3 days. They found that the EPSP usually returned to baseline levels before the population spike measure, and that in one animal the population spike was still potentiated 16 weeks after stimulation. Conversely, in examples in the rat reported by Douglas and Goddard, the EPSP remained potentiated 2 months after LTP whereas the population spike had declined to baseline levels [8].

In a systematic study of LTP duration, Barnes [57] found that the half-time of the decay of the potentiated EPSP in unanesthetized free-moving rats was 3 days, extending to 3 weeks after repeated stimulation. In accord with the findings of Douglas and Goddard [8], it was reported that population spike potentiation decayed at a faster rate than the EPSP potentiation. These experiments, however, did not use nonpotentiated control animals to test for time-dependent baseline changes, so we cannot discount the possibility that there may have been a gradual increase in the baseline responses of these animals masking a concurrent decay in the potentiated waveform.

In a more rigorous study of perforant path–granule cell LTP decay, Racine et al. [4] found that EPSP decay could best be fitted by two exponential curves with time constants of approximately 2 h and of 4.3 days, giving a half-decay time of approximately 4.5 days (estimated from their data). In contrast to the findings of Barnes and of Douglas and Goddard, but in agreement with those of Bliss and Gardner-Medwin, Racine et al. found that the EPSP decayed at a faster rate than the population spike. de Jonge and Racine also followed LTP decay for several weeks and found that all responses decayed to baseline levels over a range of 6–47 days with an average half-decay time of 13 days [58].

Although several studies appear to demonstrate that the LTP trace decays within a few weeks after stimulation, there is a methodological problem that needs to be considered when assessing this work. When electrodes are chronically located in the brain and potentials are recorded over long periods of time, there is a high probability of some electrode movement due to brain or skull changes. The standard procedure when inserting the recording electrodes into the hilus is to locate the electrode in the position where the maximum potential is recorded. It is assumed, therefore, that any shift in electrode position will lead to a reduction in the amplitude of the potential, thus avoiding the possibility of overestimating the durability of LTP. Animals showing abrupt changes are discarded, but animals showing gradual reduction of the responses will not be discarded. The results, therefore, may have a bias towards underestimation of the durability of the LTP.

At face value, however, the results show that LTP does not last indefinitely. Repetition of LTP-inducing stimulation may be required to produce permanent LTP, in much the same way that multiple experiences of a behavioral situation will improve the memory of it [58]. Although repetitive application of stimulation trains on different days has been shown to maintain LTP levels [8], the rate of decay after the final stimulation has been found to vary in different studies. de Jonge and Racine observed the same rate of decay whether only one or several repetitions of the train had been administered [58], whereas others have found more prolonged LTP if repetition is increased [2,8,57]. All studies agree that decay is observed, regardless of the conditions of induction. Taken together, the results indicate that LTP might be maintained indefinitely only if some sort of "refresh mechanism" periodically reactivates the potentiated synapses [58].

We have described how, during LTP, the EPSP and population spike components of the evoked waveform increase in uncorrelated fashion and subsequently decay at different rates, implying that the synaptic and cellular components of LTP are separable. Analysis of EPSP–population spike relationships before and after the induction of LTP provides support for this dichotomy. For example, Figure 5 shows examples of the potential evoked by stimulation of the medial perforant path (mpp) before and after LTP-inducing stimulation. The EPSP recorded before LTP induction has been matched with the EPSP recorded after LTP by adjusting the stimulus strength. For an equivalent synaptic input, a larger population spike (more cells discharging) was observed after the induction of LTP.

If the population spike height is plotted against the EPSP slope over an appropriate range of stimulus intensities (Fig. 6), creating an input/output (I/O) curve both before and after LTP-inducing stimulation, the relationship exhibits both a shift to the left and a decrease in slope. The shift to the left reflects the larger population spike per EPSP, as if there had been an increase in granule cell excitability. In this chapter it will be referred to as the "excitability shift," although we will discuss later how it might be accounted for in synaptic terms. The decrease in slope of the I/O curve may reflect an additional superimposed nonlinear decrease in excitability mediated through a separate mechanism. Abraham and Goddard [59] suggest that this separate mechanism may be LTP of perforant path connections onto feed-forward inhibitory interneurons and thus this change will be referred to as "potentiation of feed-forward inhibition." This suggestion receives support from Kairiss et al. [60], who show that if the LTP of the perforant path–granule cell connection is blocked, as described earlier, by the phenomenon of concurrent commissural stimulation [53] allowing the postulated perforant path–inhibitory interneuron synapses to be potentiated, then the subsequent lasting reduction in granule cell excitability is exaggerated.

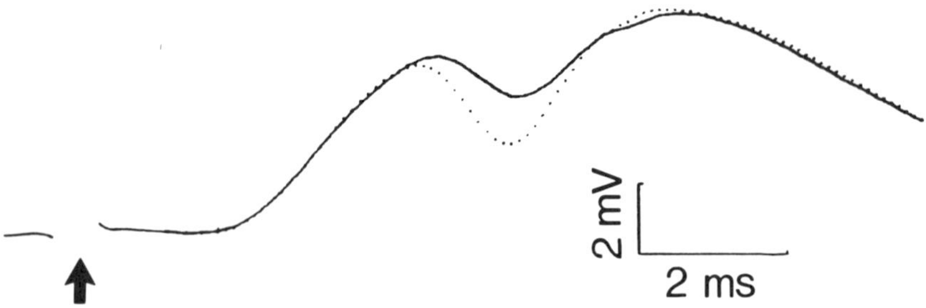

Fig. 5. Waveforms recorded before (solid line) and after (dotted line) LTP-inducing stimulation as in Figure 3. In this case the intensity of the post-LTP test pulse (arrow) is reduced so that the slope of the EPSPs are matched. Note the increase in population spike for a given EPSP after LTP.

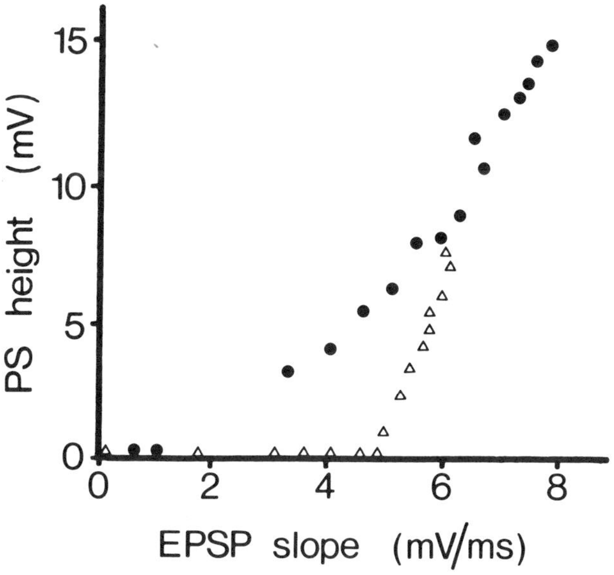

Fig. 6. Graph showing population spike height plotted against EPSP slope over a range of stimulus intensities, before (△) and after (●) LTP induction. Note the shift to the left and decrease in slope of the post-LTP function, indicating an alteration in the translation of synaptic drive to cellular activity.

2.6 Mechanisms

The finding that commissural stimulation has such marked control over perforant path LTP has important implications for theories of LTP mechanism. Its ability to block perforant path LTP indicates that the locus of control for LTP is postsynaptic, since the terminal field of the commissural afferents is too far away from the terminal field of the perforant path afferents, and the time course of their interaction in the control of LTP is too short for this interaction to be mediated extracellularly [53]. It is important to differentiate here between the location of the LTP effect itself and the location of the control mechanism. There is a body of research that suggests that the LTP mechanism is located postsynaptically. For example, Baudry and Lynch propose that LTP is the result of an increased number of postsynaptic receptors for glutamate, the putative, relevant excitatory neurotransmitter [61]. They have reported that the number of glutamate-binding sites is 30% greater in fractions prepared from hippocampal slices subjected to high-frequency stimulation than in fractions from control slices [62], and that excitatory amino acid antagonists block

LTP induction [11]. Conflicting results, however, have been obtained in other studies, which report that glutamate binding is not increased after LTP [63] and that the response of pyramidal cells to iontophoretically applied glutamate is not enhanced after LTP induction [64]

Other studies implicate a presynaptic factor in the LTP mechanism. Skrede and Malthe-Sorenssen found that high-frequency stimulation of CA1 afferents was accompanied by a long-lasting increase in the release of labeled aspartate [65], and several investigators have demonstrated that LTP is associated with a long-term increase in the release of excitatory transmitter [66–69]. Bliss et al., using a push-pull cannula technique, have reported that this increased release did not occur in the dentate gyrus when the LTP-producing effects of high-frequency stimulation were blocked by concurrent inhibition obtained by tetanization of the commissural afferents [69].

Most theories of LTP mechanism acknowledge the importance of calcium. It has been demonstrated that LTP cannot be induced in a slice preparation in which the tissue is bathed in a low calcium medium [11,70], while high levels of extracellular calcium have been shown to produce LTP in the absence of high-frequency stimulation [71,72]. Lynch et al. reported that the intracellular injection of EGTA, a substance that buffers intracellular calcium, blocked LTP induction [73], and Baimbridge and Miller have reported that calcium uptake into hippocampal slices is increased for at least 30 min after high-frequency stimulation in the CA1 area [74]. The results of these studies indicate that elevated intracellular levels of calcium are an important factor in LTP induction.

A further distinction must be made between the initiating factor or "trigger" for LTP, and the factor that sustains it over time. It appears that calcium influx is an important trigger in the process, but several theories have implicated other factors in the maintenance of LTP. For example, it has been demonstrated that N-methyl-D-aspartate (NMDA) antagonists block the induction of LTP in the slice preparation without affecting synaptic transmission [75–77]. It has been suggested that the activation of the NMDA receptors is a key element in LTP induction [76]. However, work by Sastry et al. suggests that NMDA antagonists may actually enhance long-term depression, masking the induction of LTP that occurs unaffected by the drug [78,79]. Lynch and Baudry have suggested that a postsynaptic mechanism is involved, in which calcium influx activates a proteinase that degrades a protein involved in the regulation of the shape of dendritic spines [16]. Thus this process provides a means by which high-frequency activation could lead to a change in dendritic ultrastructure, causing corresponding changes in synaptic efficacy.

It has been suggested that LTP may involve both presynaptic and postsynaptic components [15]. In one such hypothetical mechanism, a trophic substance is released from the postsynaptic region after the influx of calcium ions that accompanies a large depolarizing event. This trophic substance is fed back to presynaptic receptors and initiates the increase in transmitter release that maintains LTP. In this model, it should be possible to induce LTP by postsynaptic depolarization and to block it with subsynaptic hyperpolarization. Although Kuhnt [80] has reported that repetitive high-frequency intracellular current injection can induce LTP-type changes that last for at least 3 h, Wigstrom et al. have found that intracellular hyperpolarization does not block LTP [55]. Evidence for or against the trophic molecule aspect of the model has not been brought forward.

3 MORPHOLOGICAL CORRELATES OF LTP

3.1 Synaptic Morphology

The change in synaptic efficacy of LTP may be mediated through one or more of a variety of mechanisms, some involving morphological alterations in synaptic structure, such as an increase in the number of synapses or the structural modification of dendritic spines. With respect to the latter mechanism, several studies using mathematical models have demonstrated that a change in the shape or the electrical properties of dendritic spines could produce marked changes in synaptic efficacy [81–83]. For example, assuming passive membrane properties, spine synapses should activate the cell less well than shaft synapses [81]. In support of such models, a relationship between synapse morphology and physiological characteristics has recently been demonstrated in a sense organ of the thornback ray, *Platyrhinoides triseriata* [84]. Because of the possibility that such changes might be visualized by electron microscopy (EM) techniques, several studies have been conducted to determine whether morphological changes accompany LTP.

The methodological considerations in such studies include several important control procedures. Electrographic recording during the application of the LTP-inducing stimulation should be employed to ensure that seizures are not generated, as these might have morphological consequences quite unrelated to LTP. The LTP should be verified electrophysiologically before the tissue is prepared for morphometry, and it is important that the verification be conducted at least 10–15 min after stimulation to avoid confusion between LTP and short-duration forms of potentiation. Controls for implantation and the effects of electrical stimulation should be included, to rule out the possibility that any observed change does not result from merely placing an electrode into afferent fibers or applying low-frequency, nonpotentiating stimulation.

Several early investigations had reported changes in the synaptic morphology of peripheral nervous system structures after long-duration high-frequency stimulation of afferent fibers. Illis [85] reported an increase in terminal bouton size at up to 90 min after stimulation of a single posterior root at 300 Hz for 65 min, and Pysh and Wiley [86] found that presynaptic endings of the superior cervical ganglion developed larger contact zones and had fewer vesicles and a greater circumference after 20- to 32-Hz stimulation was applied for a period of 150–190 min. However, in these studies the synapse was not monitored electrophysiologically during or after stimulation, so it is not clear whether potentiation was induced in the preparation. Further, the application of stimulation for such extended periods of time may have induced additional changes unrelated to LTP.

The first studies of synaptic morphology conducted with specific reference to LTP were those of van Harreveld and Fifkova [87], who stimulated in mice the medial and lateral entorhinal cortex, the area of origin of the perforant path fibers, at a frequency of 30 Hz for a duration of 30 sec. They compared the morphology of the proximal third of the dentate gyrus molecular layer with that of the distal two thirds, the region where the perforant path fibers synapse. Tissue was prepared for EM by a freeze substitution process after a delay of 2–60 min after stimulation. This particular fixation procedure was chosen in an attempt to reduce the electrolyte changes caused by aldehyde fixation, which would result in volume changes in the dendrites and spines [88]. In a series of studies using these procedures [87–90] these investigators have consistently reported an increase of up to 38% in the area of dendritic spines, and a decrease in spine number in the region of the molecular layer receiving the perforant path input. The increase in spine area was initially due to an increase in the width of both the spine stalk and the spine head (tested 4 min after stimulation). When tested at longer intervals, however, only the spine head remained significantly enlarged [88].

The disadvantages of the freeze substitution method of fixation are that 1) tissue is taken from a very limited area of the quick-frozen sample, as only tissue within 10–15 μm of the cold source is suitable for EM; tissue taken from outside this area will contain artificially induced variation in morphology [87]; 2) this process cannot be applied to a structure whose integrity has been disturbed by a recording electrode, preventing either the verification of LTP or the elimination of the possibility that the tissue had experienced seizure activity. An additional problem was that van Harreveld and Fifkova took their control tissue from animals that had not received implantation or electrical stimulation and therefore one cannot be certain that the swollen dendritic spines were specifically LTP-related.

Desmond and Levy [91] also searched for morphological changes in the dentate gyrus molecular layer of rats after stimulation of the perforant path. Tissue was prepared for analysis at both 10- and 60-min intervals after stimulation. Aldehyde fixation techniques were utilized and, for the purpose of analysis, the molecular layer was divided into six separate regions, from the most proximal to the most distal to the granular layer. These investigators reported that in the principal area of synaptic activation (as tested by current source density analysis) there was a significant decrease in the numbers of small synapses observed, and an 81% increase in the number of large concave, or "cup shaped," synapses. They reported an overall increase in shaft synapses of 46%. However, this was mainly confined to the regions on the periphery of the level of maximum synaptic activation, as there was a nonsignificant decrease in this central zone. Control for the effects of electrical stimulation was achieved by analyzing hippocampal tissue from the untetanized hemisphere, which had been stimulated with low-frequency, nonpotentiating pulses. These results may give partial support to the findings of van Harreveld and Fifkova [87], at least in the sense that an increase in the number of large synapses would be consistent with a report of dendritic spine swelling.

There have also been several studies of LTP-related morphological changes in the CA1 region of the hippocampus. Lee et al. [92,93] stimulated the schaffer collateral/commissural input to area CA1 in rats. LTP induction was verified, control animals were stimulated with low-frequency stimulation trains, and aldehyde fixation techniques were used. Significant changes in morphology were associated with LTP in both intact animals and in *ex vivo* hippocampal slices tested 10–15 min after stimulation. These changes included an increase of 33–50% in the number of axodendritic shaft synapses, an increase in the ratio of shaft-to-spine synapses, and a reduction in the variability of the area of dendritic spines, the length of postsynaptic densities on spines, and the width of spine stalks. It should be noted, however, that the large percentage increase in axoshaft synapses is among a very small initial population where 96–97% of all synapses are axospinous.

A methodological problem with this study was that control and LTP preparations received unequal numbers of stimulation pulses and that changes were not monitored for periods of longer than 15 min. Chang and Greenough [94] have since attempted better control by studying synaptic morphology after inducing physiologically verified LTP in area CA1 of *ex vivo* slices of rat hippocampus. The preparations were monitored for up to 8 h after stimulation and experimental slices were compared to control slices that received the same number of electrical pulses, but at a lower, nonpotentiating frequency. It was verified that the high-frequency stimulation (300 pulses at 100 Hz) produced a 300% increase in the pyramidal cell population spike (the EPSP was not measured), tested 10–15 min after stimulation. Tissue fixation was by glutaraldehyde.

In accord with the findings of Desmond and Levy and Lee et al., Chang and Greenough [94] reported an LTP-associated increase in the number of axoshaft synapses (95% more than control slices) and a reduction in the coefficient of variation in spine head perimeter and area. They noted that the change in spine head perimeter lasted only 2 h and that the other changes remained undiminished between the 2-h and 8-h observation periods. Whereas Desmond and Levy had reported an increase in the number of concave or cup-shaped synapses, Chang and Greenough found that spine heads became rounder and that the percentage of cup-shaped heads was 12% lower in LTP slices than in control slices.

Included in the classification scheme of Chang and Greenough, and not used in previous studies, was the category "sessile spine synapse." This denotes the 1–2% of axodendritic synapses that are between the shaft and spine categories (Fig. 7) and would comprise a subcategory of the "simple" synapse group of Desmond and Levy. The inclusion of this

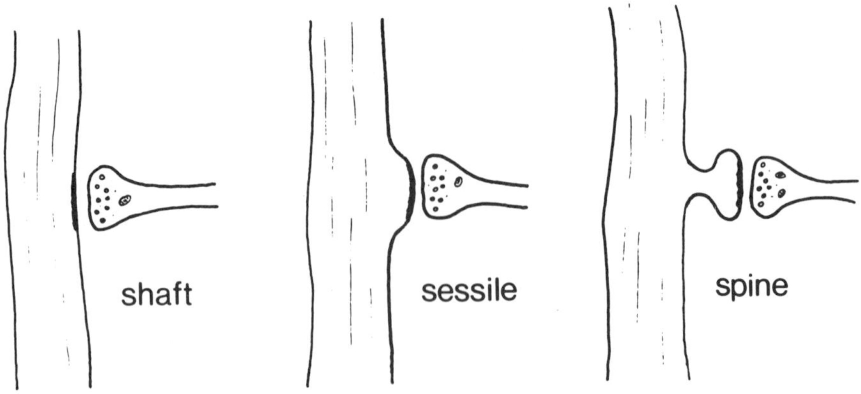

Fig. 7. Diagram illustrating examples of the shaft, sessile and spine axodendritic synapses as categorized by Chang and Greenough [94].

category appears to have allowed the recording of phenomenology previously unnoticed, as they reported a 170% increase in the number of sessile spine synapses after the induction of LTP. It is significant that both sessile and shaft synapses increase in number, as this observation provides a safeguard against the possibility that more "sessile" profiles had been classified as "shaft" in the LTP group than in the control group. No changes in any of these measures were found in slices that received either continuous high-frequency stimulation (40 or 100 Hz for 10 min) or short-duration low-frequency stimulation (300 pulses at 1 Hz).

Chang and Greenough note that the results observed would be compatible with several models of LTP mechanism. For example, a model whereby the activation of spine synapses causes a widening of the spine neck and reabsorption towards an axoshaft configuration, the opposing model where shaft synapses are the first step in a process of stimulation-induced synaptogenesis with development over time from shaft to sessile to spine synapses, or a model where spine and shaft synapses develop or atrophy independently. Unfortunately, there is no way of deciding among these hypotheses on the basis of the current morphological data.

Comparison of the results obtained from those studies conducted in area CA1 with studies conducted in the dentate gyrus reveal some interesting differences. Dentate gyrus studies report an enlargement of spine heads or more large concave synapses (quite possibly two different descriptions of the same phenomenon), and an overall increase in shaft synapses, with a nonsignificant reduction in the region of synaptic activation. By comparison CA1 studies report a decrease in the number of concave spines with an increase in shaft and sessile spine synapses. Although it has been suggested that different LTP mechanisms may exist in these two areas [94], the observed morphological differences may be due to differences in experimental techniques or differences in the dentate gyrus and CA1 neuropil.

3.2 Interpretation of Morphological Data

Since the most consistently found correlate of LTP is the increase in number of shaft and sessile synapses, we can consider how the magnitude of these changes relates to the magnitude of the physiological changes observed during LTP. Both Chang and Greenough and Desmond and Levy report that shaft synapses constitute only 3–4% of the total number of synapses and sessile synapses make up a further 1–2%, these two categories therefore making up approximately 5% of the synapses in the neuropil studied. If shaft and sessile synapses participate proportionally with the more numerous spine synapses in the generation of the field EPSP, then it seems unlikely that the relatively large physiological changes observed after LTP (often an increase in EPSP slope of more than 50% [4]) are related solely to the morphological changes observed in 5% of synapses, even if these were to double in number.

The morphological changes, however, may be related to other aspects of LTP, such as the "excitability shift." A possible consideration here is that LTP may involve several zones: a small central zone with a decreased number of shaft synapses (as reported by Desmond and Levy) and a zone peripheral to the active LTP sites receiving an increase in shaft synapses (as reported by Desmond and Levy and perhaps consistent with the findings of Lee et al. and of Chang and Greenough). The physiological implications would depend very much on the relative proportions of these two zones, and may have implications for the phenomenon of heterosynaptic depression [12–14], as well as the excitability shift.

Further analysis of the dimensions of the dendrites onto which shaft synapses occur suggests that a differentiation may be made between the shaft and sessile components of the morphological changes. Chang and Greenough note that the LTP-related increase in shaft synapses occurs not only on dendrites of less than 1 μm diameter but also on dendrites of greater than 2 μm diameter. By contrast, the increase in sessile spine synapses is primarily on dendrites of less than 2 μm diameter. The dendrites of interneurons appear to be smooth with no spines, with a diameter of greater than 2 μm, whereas in contrast, pyramidal cell dendrites are generally less than 2 μm in diameter and have spinous protrusions [95]. Chang and Greenough and Lee et al. conclude that the increase in both shaft and sessile spine synapses on small dendrites could reflect a process whereby synapses are formed on pyramidal cells, whereas the LTP-linked increase in the number of shaft synapses on large dendrites may reflect an increase in the incidence of synapses onto interneurons [93,94]. The latter change may be related to the physiological effect described earlier as the "potentiation of feed-forward inhibition."

Given the contrasting findings of studies conducted in area CA1 and the dentate gyrus, and the methodological problems of some of the earlier studies of dentate gyrus morphology, there seems to be a need for a well-controlled study of the morphological correlates of LTP in the perforant path–granule cell synapses. Such a study should include controls to determine whether the morphological changes are the product of LTP or are the result of the high-frequency stimulation *per se*. Although the results obtained by Chang and Greenough's continuous stimulation control would suggest that the latter is not the case, the definitive study would require that both control and experimental preparations receive stimulation of identical frequency and duration. To prevent both control and experimental pathways from becoming potentiated, concurrent stimulation of the "LTP-blocking" commissural input could be used in an experiment in which control and experimental preparations receive identical perforant path stimulation. Current-source-density analysis techniques [96] might be used to locate the area of maximal synaptic activation, and so guide the morphological analysis.

When analyzing changes of the type described above, it is important to be aware that the morphological changes that accompany LTP may result from, rather than cause, LTP. Correlative assumptions about their involvement in the process, however, would be an important step in the development of better theory and make possible better tests of the theory.

4 LTP AND BEHAVIOUR

In this chapter we have attempted to describe a number of the characteristics of LTP. On the basis of these characteristics it may now be appropriate to ask how well LTP matches the requirements of a memory mechanism. Although attempts have been made to correlate LTP with behavioral change [57,97], there are several methodological problems with such studies (see Morris and Baker [98] for a review). Unfortunately, from a psychological perspective several categories of memory have been defined, including long-term, short-term, iconic, working, procedural, semantic, and declarative memory (by no means a mutually exclusive or exhaustive list of the possibilities). Some of the differences between these types of memory may result from underlying variances in synaptic mechanism, but to say in what way would require an elaborate theoretical framework relating the details of behavior to the detailed structure of the brain. This framework is not available.

It is reasonable to think, however, that if experiences in the life of a rat cause LTP at certain synapses, then LTP will change the flow of neural activity on subsequent occasions. In its turn, this altered flow of neural activity will result in altered behavior. This alteration of behavior resulting from a previous experience constitutes, according to some definitions, memory. The question of importance is whether experiences in the life of the rat are likely to cause LTP. In other words, does an experience activate neurons in the entorhinal cortex in such a way that a sufficient number of neurons, converging onto the same granule cell, discharge with a polyspike burst within a short enough period of time to satisfy the rules of LTP induction?

It has been demonstrated that LTP occurs after stimulation of afferents at frequencies and durations that approximate normally occurring polyspike burst discharges, and involve an estimated coactivity of approximately 400 converging afferent fibers. Therefore, LTP in the behaving animal would require 400 layer 2 entorhinal cortex neurons, with fibers projecting to the same set of granule cells, to be active synchronously at a high frequency. The probability of such an event cannot be calculated without more detailed studies of unit recording from this area in awake animals. Such a calculation might provide strong evidence for or against the possibility that LTP has some role to play in the process of memory and learning.

5 ACKNOWLEDGMENTS

This work was supported by a grant to G.V.G. from the Medical Research Council of New Zealand. D.K.B. receives a University Grants Committee postgraduate scholarship.

6 REFERENCES

1. Cajal S Ramon y: "Histologie du systeme nerveux de l'homme et des vertebres." Paris: Moloine, 1911, Vol 2.
2. Bliss TVP, Gardner-Medwin AR: Long-lasting potentiation of synaptic transmission in the dentate area of unanesthetized rabbit following stimulation of the perforant path. J Physiol 232:357, 1973.
3. Bliss TVP, Lomo T: Long-lasting potentiation of synaptic transmission in the dentate area of the anaesthetized rabbit following stimulation of the perforant path. J Physiol 232:331, 1973.
4. Racine RJ, Milgram NW, Hafner S: Long-term potentiation phenomena in the rat limbic forebrain. Brain Res 260:217, 1983.
5. Milner B: Disorders of learning and memory after temporal lobe lesions in man. Clin Neurosurg 19:421, 1972.
6. Andersen P, Bliss TVP, Skrede KK: Lamellar organization of hippocampal excitatory pathways. Exp Brain Res 13:222, 1971.
7. Andersen P, Bliss TVP, Skrede KK: Unit analysis of hippocampal population spikes. Exp Brain Res 13:208, 1971.
8. Douglas RM, Goddard GV: Long-term potentiation of the perforant path-granule cell synapse in the rat hippocampus. Brain Res 86:205, 1975.
9. Schwartzkroin PA, Webster K: Long-lasting facilitation of a synaptic potential following tetanization in the in vitro hippocampal slice. Brain Res 89:107, 1975.
10. Anderson P, Sundberg SH, Sveen O, Wigstrom H: Specific long-term potentiation of synaptic transmission in hippocampal slices. Nature 266:736, 1977.

11. Dunwiddie T, Madison D, Lynch G: Synaptic transmission is required for initiation of long-term potentiation. Brain Res 150:413, 1978.
12. Lynch GS, Dunwiddie T, Gribkoff V: Heterosynaptic depression: A postsynaptic correlate of long-term potentiation. Nature 266:736, 1977.
13. Dunwiddie T, Lynch G: Long-term potentiation and depression of synaptic responses in the rat hippocampus: Localization and frequency dependency. J Physiol 276:353, 1978.
14. Abraham WC, Goddard GV: Asymmetric relations between homosynaptic long-term potentiation and heterosynaptic long-term depression. Nature 305:717, 1983.
15. Bliss TVP, Dolphin AC: What is the mechanism of long-term potentiation in the hippocampus? Trends Neurosci 5:289, 1982.
16. Lynch G, Baudry M: The biochemistry of memory: A new and specific hypothesis. Science 224:1057, 1984.
17. Skrede KK, Westgaard RH: The transverse hippocampal slice: A well defined cortical structure maintained in vitro. Brain Res 35:589, 1971.
18. Alger BE, Tyler TJ: Long-term and short-term plasticity in the CA1, CA3 and dentate region of the rat hippocampal slice. Brain Res 110:463, 1976.
19. Wigstrom H, Gustafsson B: Large long-lasting potentiation in the dentate gyrus in vitro during blockade of inhibition. Brain Res 275:153, 1983.
20. Laroche S, Bloch V: Conditioning of hippocampal cells and long-term potentiation: An approach to mechanisms of post-trial memory facilitation. In Ajome-Marson C, Mathies H (eds): "Biological Basis of Learning and Memory Formation." IBRO Monograph Series, Vol 9. London: Raven, 1981.
21. Bloch V, Laroche S: Enhancement of long-term potentiation in the rat dentate gyrus by post-trial stimulation of the reticular formation. J Physiol 360:215, 1985.
22. Bliss TVP, Goddard GV, Riives M: Reduction of long-term potentiation in the dentate gyrus of the rat following selective depletion of monoamines. J Physiol 334:475, 1983.
23. Robinson GB, Racine RJ: Long-term potentiation in the dentate gyrus: Effects of noradrenaline depletion in the awake rat. Brain Res 325:71, 1985.
24. Dunwiddie TV, Roberson NL, Worth T: Modulation of long-term potentiation: Effects of adrenergic and neuroleptic drugs. Pharmacol Biochem Behav 17:1257, 1982.
25. Lee KS: Sustained enhancement of evoked potentials following brief, high frequency stimulation of the cerebral cortex in vitro. Brain Res 239:617, 1982.
26. Kreig WG: Connections of the cerebral cortex. I. The albino rat. A topography of the cortical areas. J Comp Neurol 84:221, 1946.
27. Baranyi A, Feher O: Synaptic facilitation requires paired activation of convergent pathways in the neocortex. Nature 290:413, 1981.
28. Woody CD (ed): "Conditioning: Representation of Involved Neural Functions." Advances in Behavioral Biology, Vol 26. New York: Plenum, 1982.
29. Ito M, Sakurai M, Tongroach P: Climbing fibre induced depression of both mossy fibre responsiveness and glutamate sensitivity of cerebellar purkinje cells. J Physiol 324:113, 1982.
30. Gerren RA, Weinberger NM: Long-term potentiation in the magnocellular medial geniculate nucleus of the anesthetized cat. Brain Res 265:138, 1983.
31. Brown TH, McAfee DA: Long-term synaptic potentiation in the superior cervical ganglion. Science 215:1411, 1982.
32. Briggs CA, Brown TH, McAfee DA: Neurophysiology and pharmacology of long-term potentiation in the rat sympathetic ganglion. J Physiol 359:503, 1985.

33. Skelton RW, Miller JJ, Phillips AG: Low frequency stimulation of the perforant path produces long-term potentiation in the dentate gyrus of unanaesthetized rats. Can J Physiol Pharmacol 61:1156, 1983.
34. Barrionuevo G, Schottler F, Lynch G: The effects of repetitive low-frequency stimulation on control and 'potentiated' synaptic responses in the hippocampus. Life Sci 27:2358, 1980.
35. Goddard GV, McIntyre DC, Leech C: A permanent change in brain function resulting from daily electrical stimulation. Exp Neurol 25:295, 1969.
36. Goddard GV, Douglas RM: Does the engram of kindling model the engram of normal long-term memory. Can J Neurol Sci 2:385, 1975.
37. Racine R, Newberry F, Burnham WM: Post-activation potentiation and the kindling phenomenon. Electroencephalogr Clin Neurophysiol 39:261, 1975.
38. Douglas RM: Temporal characteristics of stimuli that produce long-term potentiation. In Fehér O, Joó F (eds): "Cellular Analogues of Conditioning." Oxford: Pergamon, 1981, p 187.
39. Vinogradova OS: Functional organization of the limbic system in the process of registration of information: Facts and hypothesis. In Isaacson RL, Pribram KH (eds): "The Hippocampus, Vol 2." New York: Plenum, 1975, p 26.
40. Hebb DO: "The Organisation of Behavior." New York: Wiley Interscience, 1949.
41. McNaughton BL, Douglas RM, Goddard GV: Synaptic enhancement in fascia dentate: Cooperativity among coactive afferents. Brain Res 157:277, 1978.
42. Wigstrom H, Gustafsson B: Heterosynaptic modulation of homosynaptic long-lasting potentiation in the hippocampal slice. Acta Physiol Scand 119:455, 1983.
43. Levy WB, Steward O: Synapses as associative memory elements in the hippocampal formation. Brain Res 175:233, 1979.
44. Levy WB, Steward O: Temporal contiguity requirements for long-term associative potentiation/depression in the hippocampus. Neuroscience 8:791, 1983.
45. Lee KS: Cooperativity among afferents for the induction of long-term potentiation in the CA1 region of the hippocampus. J Neurosci 3:1369, 1983.
46. Kelso SR, Brown TH: Temporal contiguity requirements for associative long-term potentiation in hippocampal slices. Soc Neurosci Abstr 10:78, 1984.
47. Fantie BD: Augmentation of dentate granule cell population spikes after high frequency trains delivered to the septum and perforant path. Soc Neurosci Abstr 8:315, 1982.
48. Robinson GB, Racine RJ: Heterosynaptic interactions between septal and entorhinal inputs to the dentate gyrus: Long-term potentiation effects. Brain Res 249:162, 1982.
49. Bilkey DK: High frequency medial septal stimulation activates perforant path fibres. Proc Univ Otago Med School 63:3, 1985.
50. Bilkey DK, Goddard GV: Medial septal facilitation of hippocampal granule cell activity is mediated by inhibition of inhibitory interneurons. Brain Res (in press).
51. McNaughton BL, Barnes CA, Anderson P: Synaptic efficacy and EPSP summation in granule cells of rat fascia dentate studied in vitro. J Neurophysiol 46:952, 1981.
52. Braitenburg V, Schuz A: Some anatomical comments on the hippocampus. In Seifert W (ed): "Neurobiology of the Hippocampus." London: Academic, 1983, p 31.
53. Douglas RM, Goddard GV, Riives M: Inhibitory modulation of long-term potentiation: Evidence for a postsynaptic locus of control. Brain Res 240:259, 1982.
54. Douglas RM, McNaughton BL, Goddard GV: Commissural inhibition and facilitation of granule cell discharge in fascia dentata. J Comp Neurol 219:285, 1983.

55. Wigstrom H, McNaughton BL, Barnes CA: Long-term synaptic enhancement in hippocampus is not regulated by postsynaptic membrane potential. Brain Res 233:195, 1982.
56. Scharfman HE, Sarvey JM: Postsynaptic firing during repetitive stimulation is required for long-term potentiation in hippocampus. Brain Res 331:267, 1985.
57. Barnes CA: Memory deficits associated with senescence: A behavioral and neurophysiological study in the rat. J Comp Physiol Psychol 93:74, 1979.
58. de Jonge M, Racine R: The effects of repeated induction of long-term potentiation in the dentate gyrus. Brain Res 328:181, 1985.
59. Abraham WC, Goddard GV: Multiple traces of neural activity in the hippocampus. In Lynch G, McGaugh JL, Weinberger NM (eds): "Neurobiology of Learning and Memory, Vol 2." New York: Guilford (in press).
60. Kairiss, EW, Abraham, WC Goddard, GV: Brain Res (in press).
61. Baudry M, Lynch G: Hypothesis regarding the cellular mechanisms responsible for long-term synaptic potentiation in the hippocampus. Exp Neurol 68:202, 1980.
62. Baudry M, Oliver M, Creager R, Wieraszko A, Lynch G: Increase in glutamate receptors following repetitive electrical stimulation in hippocampal slices. Life Sci 27:325, 1980.
63. Sastry BR, Goh JW: Long-lasting potentiation in hippocampus is not due to an increase in glutamate receptors. Life Sci 34:1497, 1984.
64. Lynch GS, Gribkoff V, Deadwyler SA: Long-term potentiation is accompanied by a reduction in dendritic responsiveness to glutamic acid. Nature 263:151, 1976.
65. Skrede KK, Malthe-Sorenssen D: Increased resting and evoked release of transmitter following repetitive electrical tetanization in hippocampus: A biochemical correlate to long-lasting synaptic potentiation. Brain Res 208:436, 1981.
66. Voronin LL: Cellular mechanisms of long-term posttetanic potentiation in the hippocampus. Adv Physiol Sci 36:165, 1980.
67. Dolphin AC, Errington ML, Bliss TVP: Long-term potentiation of the perforant path in vivo is associated with increased glutamate release. Nature 297:496, 1982.
68. Lynch M, Errington ML, Bliss TVP: Sustained increase in release of endogenous glutamate associated with long-term potentiation of the perforant path in the anaesthetized rat. Neurosci Lett Suppl 18:194, 1984.
69. Bliss TVP, Douglas RM, Errington ML, Lynch M: Correlation between release of endogenous glutamate and long-term potentiation in the dentate gyrus of anaesthetized rats. J Physiol 361:50P, 1984.
70. Dunwiddie TV, Lynch G: The relationship between extracellular calcium concentrations and the induction of hippocampal long-term potentiation. Brain Res 169:103, 1979.
71. Bliss TVP, Dolphin AC, Feasey KJ: Elevated calcium induces a long-lasting potentiation of commissural responses in hippocampal CA3 cells of the rat in vivo. J Physiol 350:65P, 1984.
72. Turner RW, Baimbridge KG, Miller JJ: Calcium-induced long-term potentiation in the hippocampus. Neuroscience 7:1411, 1982.
73. Lynch G, Larson J, Kelso S, Barrionuevo G, Schottler F: Intracellular injections of EGTA block induction of hippocampal long-term potentiation. Nature 305:719, 1983.
74. Baimbridge KG, Miller JJ: Calcium uptake and retention during long-term potentiation of neuronal activity in the rat hippocampal slice preparation. Brain Res 221:299, 1981.

75. Collingridge GL, Kehl SJ, McLennan H: Excitatory amino acids in synaptic transmission in the schaffer collateral-commissural pathway of the rat hippocampus. J Physiol 334:33, 1983.
76. Harris EW, Ganong AH, Cotman CW: Long-term potentiation in the hippocampus involves activation of N-methyl-D-aspartate receptors. Brain Res 323:132, 1984.
77. Wigstrom H, Gustafsson B: A possible correlate of the postsynaptic condition for long-lasting potentiation in the guinea pig hippocampus in vitro. Neurosci Lett 44:327, 1984.
78. Sastry BR, Chirwa SS, Goh JW, Maretic H, Pandanaboina MM: Verapamil counteracts depression but not long-term potentiation of the hippocampal population spike. Life Sci 34:1075, 1984.
79. Sastry BR, Goh JW, Pandanaboina MM: Verapamil counteracts the masking of long-term potentiation of hippocampal population spike produced by 2-amino-5-phosphonovalerate. Life Sci 34:323, 1984.
80. Kuhnt U: Long-lasting changes of synaptic excitability induced by repetitive intracellular current injections in hippocampal neurons. Neurosci Lett Suppl 18:S27, 1984.
81. Rall W: Cable properties of dentrites and effects of synaptic location. In Anderson P, Jansen JKS (eds): "Excitatory Synaptic Mechanisms." Oslo: Universitetsforlaget, 1970, p 175.
82. Miller JP, Rall W, Rinzel J: Synaptic amplification by active membrane in dendritic spines. Brain Res 325:325, 1985.
83. Perkel DH, Perkel DJ: Dendritic spines: Role of active membrane in modulating synaptic efficacy. Brain Res 325:331, 1985.
84. Fields DR, Ellisman MH: Synaptic morphology and differences in sensitivity. Science 228:197, 1985.
85. Illis LS: Enlargement of spinal cord synapses after repetitive stimulation of the single posterior root. Nature 223:76, 1969.
86. Pysh JJ, Wiley RG: Morphological alterations of synapses in electrically stimulated superior cervical ganglia of the cat. Science 176:191, 1972.
87. van Harreveld A, Fifkova E: Swelling of dendritic spines in the fascia dentata after stimulation of the perforant fibres as a mechanism of post-tetanic potent. Exp Neurol 49:736, 1975.
88. Fifkova E, Anderson CL: Stimulation induced changes in the dimensions of stalks of dendritic spines in the dentate molecular layer. Exp Neurol 74:621, 1981.
89. Fifkova E, Anderson CL, Young SJ, van Harreveld A: Effect of anisomycin on stimulation-induced changes in the dendritic spines of the dentate granule cells. J Neurocytol 11:183, 1982.
90. Fifkova E, van Harreveld A: Long-lasting morphological changes in dendritic spines of dentate granular cells following stimulation of the entorhinal area. J Neurocytol 6:211, 1977.
91. Desmond NL, Levy WB: Synaptic correlates of associative potentiation/depression: An ultrastructural study in the hippocampus. Brain Res 265:21, 1983.
92. Lee K, Oliver M, Schottler F, Creager R, Lynch G: Ultrastructural effects of repetitive stimulation in the hippocampal slice preparation: A preliminary report. Exp Neurol 65:478, 1979.
93. Lee KS, Schottler MO, Lynch G: Brief bursts of high frequency stimulation produce two types of structural change in rat hippocampus. J Neurophysiol 44:247, 1980
94. Chang FLF, Greenough WT: Transient and enduring morphological correlates of synaptic activity and efficacy change in the rat hippocampal slice. Brain Res 309:35, 1984.

95. Anderson P, Gross GN, Lomo T, Sveen O: Participation of inhibitory and excitatory interneurons in the control of hippocampal cortical output. In Brazier, M (ed): "The Interneuron." Los Angeles: University of California Press, 1969, p 417.
96. Nicholson C: Theoretical analysis of field potentials in anisotropic ensembles of neuronal elements. IEEE Trans Biomed Eng 20:278, 1973.
97. Berger TLW: Long-term potentiation of hippocampal synaptic transmission affects rate of behavioural learning. Science 224:627, 1984.
98. Morris R, Baker M: Does long-term potentiation/synaptic enhancement have anything to do with learning or memory? In Squire LR, Butters N (eds): "The Neuropsychology of memory." New York: Guildford, 1984.

2

Effects of Ethanol on Synaptic Membrane Biochemistry During the Brain Growth Spurt

Elizabeth M. Burns

This review highlights the potential dangers of ethanol exposure of relatively low intensity and short duration during synaptogenesis. Previously, the major emphasis of studies on the effects of alcohol during brain ontogeny has been focused primarily on the effects of alcoholism *per se*. However, the high risk to infants born of alcoholic women and the devastating effects of the fetal alcohol syndrome (FAS) have demanded investigation of FAS-related problems. The heightened susceptibility of rapidly developing synaptic structures during the brain growth spurt, the subtle though serious damage that may result from lower-intensity and shorter-duration ethanol exposure during that time period, the increasing frequency of moderate to heavy social drinking in our society, and evidence that birth weight is significantly lowered in the offspring of women consuming one or two drinks per day, underline the need for studies on the effects of ethanol during synaptogenesis. Although exposure of the brain to blood ethanol concentrations associated with social or binge drinking is not expected to have the devastating effects of alcoholism, it may nevertheless compromise the quality of life of affected individuals. In this review a number of developmental issues are discussed. These include the existence of vulnerable periods during brain ontogeny, the sequence of events occurring during synaptogenesis, the properties of developing pre- and postsynaptic membranes, and the mechanisms involved in recognition and adhesion processes implicated in the establishment of synaptic connectivity. These provide a background for appreciating the potentially damaging effects of alcohol, which is known to perturb membrane structure and function even in the mature animal. Also reviewed are the problems that have hampered alcohol studies in neonatal animals. An animal model is proposed, and findings from studies using this animal model are described. Because of the potential dangers of relatively low blood ethanol concentrations during the brain growth spurt, some recent clinical uses of ethanol are also reviewed.

From the College of Nursing, The University of Iowa, Iowa City, Iowa 52242, USA.

Current Topics in Research on Synapses, Volume 3, pages 29–76 **© 1986 Alan R. Liss, Inc.**

1 INTRODUCTION

Maternal ethanol intake during pregnancy is detrimental to human fetal development [1–7]. It is now well documented that the offspring of alcoholic mothers are at risk of manifesting the fetal alcohol syndrome (FAS), a constellation of developmental anomalies first given world attention in 1973 by Jones and Smith [1]. The main characteristics of the FAS are pre- and postnatal growth deficiency, microcephaly, characteristic facial features, limb and organ anomalies, and behavioral disorders.

1.1 Incidence of FAS

In a review of the FAS and its neurological sequelae, Colangelo and Jones [8] stated that the incidence of FAS in the general population, as reported in the literature, varied between 0.4 and 3.1 per 1,000 live births. However, the incidence of FAS in infants born of chronically alcoholic women has been found to be 24 per 1,000 [9], 25 per 1,000 [10], or 29 per 1,000 [11]. Furthermore, to date, the full FAS has been observed only in infants born to chronically intoxicated women, e.g. women whose daily ethanol intake is equal to or greater than six drinks per day.

1.2 Subtle Deficits

The full spectrum of neuropsychological defects thought to be related to ethanol exposure during human brain ontogeny ranges in severity from the mental retardation associated with the FAS to the more subtle though serious abnormalities of attention deficit disorder [12] and hyperactivity [13]. The severity of ethanol-induced neuropsychological deficits depends undoubtedly on the timing, intensity, and duration of the exposure, and on various other factors including genetic sensitivity, interactions with other drugs, and the nutritional status of the mother. Deficits at the synaptic molecular level are less easily identified than are gross neuropathological deficits, and yet these too may interfere with neurological function.

2 VULNERABLE PERIODS

The more rapid the rate of growth of an organ or a tissue, the greater is its vulnerability. Three phases of mammalian neuroontogeny have been identified as being particularly susceptible to injury by teratogenic agents. These are organogenesis, rapid neuronal proliferation, and the brain growth spurt. However, different systems within the brain develop at different times during ontogeny and each system develops at its own rate. In general, the development of the central nervous system (CNS) proceeds in a sequential caudocranial manner [14]. Maturation of the spinal cord is followed by that of the myelencephalon, mesencephalon, diencephalon, and telencephalon [15]. The cerebellum has attracted much attention relative to its postnatal development [16–20]. Del Cerro and Snider [21] found that postnatal cerebellar development does not proceed at a continuous rate but is characterized by waves of mitotic activity and cell migration separated by waves of less intense activity. They observed accelerated cerebellar maturation in the rat during days postnatal 1–3, 9–12, and 16–

19. Their observations of cerebellar growth are in keeping with findings relative to growth of the whole brain in rodents [22]. Three discrete phases of rapid growth within the brain growth spurt were found to occur during days 0–6, 8–12, and 17–23. Thus, during any specific time frame, exposure to a teratogen may selectively and significantly affect brain regions, systems, or parts of systems that are the most vulnerable at the time of exposure.

2.1 Organogenesis

Organogenesis, a time of critical vulnerability for the entire organism, occurs in the human during gestation weeks 3–9. Events characteristic of this developmental phase include establishment of the basic embryonic plan of the brain and induction of the various parts of the future central and peripheral nervous systems. These events are mediated by fundamental cellular mechanisms: proliferation, migration, differentiation, and cellular death. The effects of teratogenic agents during organogenesis are likely to be devastating, either causing embryonal death or major morphological abnormalities [23]. Also, increased mortality in children born of alcoholic mothers might be anticipated. Jones et al. [3] reported 17% perinatal mortality in offspring of alcoholic women, compared with 2% in offspring of nonalcoholic women. Neither is the finding of gross neuropathology surprising in infants born of alcoholic women. Clarren et al. [5] observed neuroglial heterotopias, dysplasias, and ectopic disorganized neuronal arrangements in histological studies of infants who died perinatally and whose mothers were chronic alcoholics. It was thought that the neuropathology in the midbrain and cerebellum in these infants had resulted from injury prior to 45 days after conception and that in the cerebrum was thought to have been induced by injury that had occurred at least by 85 days after conception [24].

2.2 Rapid Neuronal Proliferation

A second vulnerable period in human brain ontogeny occurs during gestation weeks 12–20 [25]. This period encompasses the most rapid phase of neuronal mitotic activity. Because of the rapid rate of cellular proliferation at this time, the entire developing nervous system is particularly susceptible to injury. However, there is a paucity of information concerning the effects of teratogens during this time frame.

2.3 Brain Growth Spurt

The final vulnerable period for the developing human brain begins early in the last trimester of pregnancy and continues throughout the first

18–24 months after birth. This time period in the human encompasses the most rapid phase of brain growth and is known as the brain growth spurt. Because of the rapidity of its growth the brain is extremely susceptible to teratogenic agents during this developmental phase. Thus it is likely that a lower intensity and/or a shorter duration of exposure to a teratogen during the brain growth spurt may cause brain damage. Regardless of species, or of its timing with respect to birth, the brain growth spurt is characterized by dendritic arborization, axonal growth, peak synaptogenesis, gliogenesis, myelination, and the maturation of receptors, neurotransmitters, and neurotransmission [26–28].

3 SYNAPTOGENESIS

Any of the events that occur during the brain growth spurt may be affected deleteriously by the presence of teratogens. Because of the key role of the synapse in the maintenance of the integrity of the entire nervous system, synaptic events are of particular interest. Reflection on the numerous regulatory roles of the mammalian nervous system emphasizes the importance of maintaining its integrity. It regulates autonomic functions including respiration, circulation, thermoregulation, and digestion; it also controls motor function, and governs perception, emotion, cognition, introspection, learning, memory, and behavior. Integrity of synapses is essential to information processing in the complex vertebrate nervous system. Together, synapses and neurotransmitters enable interneuronal communication: the synapses provide the dynamic structural substrate and the neurotransmitters serve as agents. Whatever affects the molecular structural integrity of either of these, therefore, will affect neurological function.

It is well established that a variety of pharmacological agents affect neuronal and synaptic membranes in mature animals. Less information is available relative to the effects of these agents during ontogeny. During synaptogenesis, when neuronal membrane elaboration is occurring at its most rapid rate, any of these agents may subserve a teratogenic role. Interference with any of the fundamental processes involved in the establishment of synapses is likely to result in synaptic pathology at the molecular level.

3.1 Synaptic Plasticity

Although there is some evidence of plasticity in synapses [29] and in neurotransmitters [30] in the adult mammalian brain, plasticity in each of these systems is probably maximal during ontogeny. Thus the period of maximal vulnerability of developing synaptic structures would be expected to coincide with the period of maximal plasticity of these structures. Hence, if brain damage has occurred prior to birth in the human, rehabilitative efforts in early postnatal life may be effective in repair of the damage, because the period of maximal plasticity of the human brain includes the third trimester of pregnancy and the first 18–24 months after birth.

3.2 Sequential Steps in Synaptogenesis

Burry et al. [31] recently presented a sequential feedback hypothesis of synaptogenesis based on the assumption that a sequential series of events takes place during synaptogenesis. The first step in the series requires the presence of specific negatively charged groups on a region of the membrane surface that forms a growth cone capable of developing into, or destined to become, a presynaptic terminal. Simultaneously, the outer membrane surface of the future postsynaptic element contains positively charged groups capable of serving as attachment sites. The second step includes the initial recognition and adhesion mechanisms that occur between the leading edge of the growth cone and the postsynaptic attachment site. The third step initiates the formation of the future synapse including formation of the synaptic cleft, loss of the morphological characteristics of the growth cone, and enlargement of the presynaptic terminal. During the fourth step, presynaptic vesicles form, the postsynaptic density begins to develop, and receptors may be detected. In the fifth step, presynaptic vesicles increase in size and number with continued maturation of the postsynaptic density occurring. In the sixth step, synaptic cleft material becomes visible. Finally, in the seventh step, presynaptic dense projections appear and neurotransmitter release can be observed.

3.3 Absence of Functional Activity Affects Synapse Maturation

Burry et al. [31] pointed out that even after completion of the series of sequential steps, the synapse still can regress. This occurs particularly in the absence of functional activity. This is relevant for the present discussion since functional activity is depressed by ethanol. For example, in a study conducted in healthy pregnant women who were light social drinkers (one to three drinks per week) fetal breathing activity was monitored by noninvasive ultrasound techniques [32]. Breathing records of seven fetuses (34–39 weeks gestation) exposed to 31 ml of 80 proof vodka in 90 ml of artificially sweetened ginger ale were compared with those of control subjects whose mothers drank only diet ginger ale. The parameters measured were breathing rate, regularity of breathing, proportion of time spent breathing, apnea (time of onset and duration of episode), and other fetal movements. Monitoring was carried out during the 30 min prior to, and 60 min after, consumption of the beverage. Blood alcohol and glucose levels were determined prior to and after ingestion of alcohol. All of the alcohol-exposed fetuses, but none of the controls, stopped breathing within 3–31 min after maternal drinking. Blood glucose levels were not affected. The investigators interpreted the results as a direct pharmacological effect of alcohol. Since fetal breathing movements reflect neurological activity, depressed functional activity following alcohol ingestion poses a threat to the developing brain. In this context, it would be of interest to know whether light or moderate social drinking might contribute toward the etiology of the "sudden infant death syndrome."

3.4 Basis of Synaptic Teratology

The model proposed by Burry and co-workers [31] for the development of a synapse is, as pointed out by those authors, the simplest model possible. Their hypothesis states that synaptogenesis proceeds by a series of steps in which completion of a preceding step is required before the subsequent step can be initiated. Furthermore, the initiation of each step takes place only when interaction occurs between the developing pre- and postsynaptic elements. Completion of the sequence of steps in an orderly manner allows development of all the synaptic machinery required for appropriately matched synaptic elements to establish synaptic connectivity. Each step in the series may be viewed as a part of the process that determines the specificity of the developing synaptic elements. Consideration of this model should enhance understanding of the potential effects of teratogens during synaptogenesis, since under normal conditions, improperly matched synaptic elements may not proceed to the formation of a mature synapse. In the presence of teratogens, disorder is likely to be introduced, thus compromising the fine wiring of the nervous system.

For example, upon exposure to ethanol during the brain growth spurt, alterations in the molecular specificity of surface membranes as well as an increase in fluidity of future pre- and postsynaptic membranes is likely to occur. Because of the billions of developing synapses present at any one time, large numbers of synaptic structures would be undergoing each of the steps in the sequential series discussed above. Thus, the altered specificity and increased fluidity of membranes might interfere with the development of growth cones and their filopodia, with recognition and initial attachment of pre- and postsynaptic elements, or with adhesion processes between growth cones and their attachment sites on future postsynaptic elements.

4 SYNAPTIC PLASMA MEMBRANES (SPMs)

4.1 General Properties of Membranes

According to a recent description of membrane structure [33], all membranes have a common phospholipid bilayer with proteins absorbed to the surface or integrated into the lipid bilayer. The various components of the membrane (i.e., proteins, lipids, and carbohydrates) are distributed asymmetrically across the lipid bilayer. Some proteins are distributed randomly within the bilayer, but others are highly organized into specific functional patterns.

Membranes exist in a highly dynamic state and exhibit rotational and lateral diffusion of the protein and lipid components of the bilayer. The chemical composition of a membrane continuously varies as new membrane components are inserted and previous components are removed, degraded, and recycled. Movement within the membrane is controlled in part by a cytoskeleton. An important point emphasized by Robertson [34] in his hydrophobic barrier membrane model is that the core of the bilayer, even when traversed by protein, is hydrophobic.

4.2 Properties of Neuronal Membranes

The neuronal plasma membrane exhibits a trilaminar structure, 8–10 nm in width. Biochemically, it is composed of lipids (mostly phospholipids and cholesterol) and numerous types of proteins and glycoproteins [35]. A notable difference between neuronal and other biological membranes is the high concentration of gangliosides in the former. Physicochemically, the neuronal lipid bilayer is highly fluid, as in other plasma membranes. On the whole, neuronal plasma membranes are structurally, biochemically, and physicochemically similar to other eukaryotic membranes.

Both synaptosomal and axonal plasma membranes appear to be characterized by highly unsaturated, and therefore probably higher fluid, lipid phases [36]. These properties are important in the ordering of the vast network of the brain. As pointed out by Pfenninger and Maylie-Pfenninger [37], the primary ordering or organizing of the brain leads to the formation of cellular arrays and to the specific cytoarchitectonics of brain regions, nuclei, and centers. A second ordering phenomenon then links appropriate neurons and target regions. This involves guided outgrowth of neurites, recognition of appropriate target cells, and finally the establishment of synaptic connectivity. Three crucial factors contribute to this ordering process: humoral substances, the intercellular matrix, and the cell surfaces. Of these three, the most attractive as a regulator during development is the cell surface—i.e., the specialized SPM microarchitectonics. Numerous studies have shown that alteration of the chemical properties of the neuronal plasma membrane may lead to changes in cellular behavior [38].

4.3 Surface Properties of Neuronal Membranes

The neuronal cell surface represents the substrate of intercellular interaction. The fluid layer of lipids is permeated by proteins with their polar portions extended out into the hydrophilic environment of either the extracellular space or intracellular cytosol, or both [39]. The polar portions adjacent to the lipid bilayer are made up of protein and carbohydrate. The carbohydrates are linked to the glycoprotein or glycolipid molecules anchored in the membrane. In contrast to the intracellular leaflet of the membrane, the outer surface has a high carbohydrate content and negative charge. As noted by Pfenninger [35], these features are particularly striking at the synaptic cleft. Gangliosides and glycoproteins contribute significantly to the carbohydrate content as well as to the negative charge of the neuronal membrane surface.

4.4 Role of the Cell Surface in Recognition

On the basis that the cell surface is an important element in cellular recognition and developmental control mechanisms, Pfenninger and Maylie-Pfenninger [37] investigated the distribution and changes in plasmalemmal glycoconjugates (glycolipids and glycoproteins) during neuronal differentiation, using cell surface labeling with ferritin-conjugated lectins that were localized and quantified electron optically. They found that both neuronal and neural crest cells and their derivatives acquired distinctive cell surface properties while still within the neuroectoderm. As these cells further differentiated, the neuronal cell surface glycoconjugate compositions changed. However, the difference between the two cell types was maintained. Within the two classes, each neuronal type expressed its own characteristic "surface carbohydrate signature" prior to sending out axon and dendrites. As neurites formed, neurons increased their surface yet maintained their specific surface properties by localized insertion distally of preassembled membrane. Upon recognition of and adhesion to its target cell, the axonal surface glycoconjugates were altered again by a process of localized membrane differentiation normal to synaptogenesis. Pfenninger and Maylie-Pfenninger [37] then concluded that neuronal specificity or "signature" is expressed on the cell surface by its glycoconjugate pattern, indicating neuronal type and state of differentiation. These findings support the hypothesis of Barondes [40] that glycomacromolecules on neuronal surfaces mediate specific interneuronal recognition.

4.5 Axonal Neurite Plasma Membranes

Pfenninger and Rees [39] observed substantial cytochemical differences between synaptic axolemma and the plasma membrane of growth cones. Ultrastructural studies revealed intramembrane particles (IMPs) thought to represent integral membrane proteins [41]. In mature axons they observed that IMPs are uniformly distributed along the axon shaft, and in growing axons they noted a decreasing IMP density gradient in a somatofugal direction. They found regional differences with respect to IMP size. The distribution of each size class of particle formed a decreasing gradient also in the somatofugal direction. These observations are in keeping with lateral diffusion and proximal insertion of membrane components into the axonal plasma membrane [42]. However, they found the membrane composition of the growth cone to be independent of these density gradients. It displayed a mosaic pattern of discrete high and low particle densities. Based on these observations they suggested that axonal shaft and growth cone membranes are biochemically and functionally distinct. This is consistent with their lectin labeling data [43], which showed regional distribution of surface glycoconjugates on sprouting neurons. They pointed out that density gradients persisted only during axonal elongation. Thus, evidence reported by these researchers supports the view that plasmalemmal expansion during axonal growth results from distal insertion of new components probably as preformed vesicles [44,45].

In another study, Pfenninger and colleagues [46] developed a method for isolating growth cone particles. This method should enable analysis of molecular mechanisms involved in growth cone function in the establishment of synaptic connections. They also observed regional variations in transmembrane proteins that suggested differences in ion channel densities [41]. Subsequently, they found corresponding regional differences in sodium channel density in growing axons [47].

Goodman et al. [48] studied similar cellular and molecular mechanisms in the nervous system of insect embryos. They found that the growth cones of identified neurons express selective affinities for specific axonal surfaces. They suggest that, early in development, cell lineage and cell interactions lead to the differential expression of cell recognition molecules on the surfaces of small subsets of embryonic neurons whose axons selectively fasciculate with one another.

The specificities of developing SPMs are crucially important in the establishment of synaptic connectivity. For example, during the growth of the axon terminal toward the site of a future synapse, it is the specificity of arrangement of the molecular components of the leading edge of the growth cone, as well as that of the future postsynaptic membrane, that enables recognition by the axon terminal of its appropriate target site. Specificity is also involved in the process of synaptic adhesion of the developing pre- and postsynaptic elements [36]. SPM specificities involve fundamental membrane constituents that are characteristic of SPMs and that distinguish SPMs from both nonsynaptic portions of neuronal plasma membranes and from nonneuronal plasma membranes (e.g., glial membranes). Even within the synaptic region, these specificities distinguish nonjunctional from junctional regions of pre- and postsynaptic portions of SPMs. Further, these specificities are such that they enable a developing neuron of a given transmitter type to establish contact with its appropriate target on a neuron of a different transmitter type. Thus, SPM specificity determines the final position, morphology, and function of the synapse.

Babitch [49] examined the association of microtubular components with SPMs in highly purified synaptosomal membranes after depolymerization of cytoplasmic microtubules. The remaining membrane-bound tubulin could be removed only by agents that dispersed the membrane. Thus he concluded that synaptic membrane tubulin is an integral component of the membrane.

Hitzemann and Harris [50] studied developmental changes in synaptic membrane fluidity. It had previously been shown that cortical SPMs increase in apparent viscosity or decrease in fluidity during development [51]. Hitzemann and Harris [50] were able to show that the changes during development were primarily in the interior of the membrane. They pointed out that the most significant change during development in SPMs is a marked increase in the cholesterol-to-lipid-P ratio, that fatty acid unsaturation increased slightly but significantly, whereas the level of phospholipid methylation decreased significantly, and that the protein-to-lipid-P ratio increased significantly during development. Hitzemann and Harris [50] predicted that gangliosides would play a role in the developmental changes in SPM fluidity, their data supporting a small but significant decrease in fluidity at the SPM membrane surface. Cholesterol has been shown to be required for pharmacological concentrations of ethanol to affect membrane order [52]. Further, Hitzemann and Harris [50] predicted that ethanol would be less effective in perturbing SPM fluidity in developing animals than in adults because the cholesterol content in neonatal animals is approximately 50% of that in the adult. However, they found no significant age-dependent effect of ethanol on membrane fluidity. According to their data, those features of membrane organization that subserve ethanol sensitivity are already operative by day 3 after birth.

4.6 Neuron Cell-Specific Adhesion Molecules

In 1976, Edelman [38] suggested that the major problem of morphogenesis at the molecular level concerns the coordination of signals for the fundamental cellular processes that give rise to tissue and organ formation. At that time, he raised two questions: "How specific must cell-cell adhesion be in order to guarantee orderly signaling?" and "What establishes the priority of the various signals for growth, motion, or cell adhesion?" The nature of these fundamental processes must be such that they are mutually exclusive. He then proposed that transmembrane control, mediated by molecular mechanisms of surface modulation, might have the necessary properties for the regulatory role needed in recognition and adhesion processes.

Edelman and colleagues [53,54] described neural cell adhesion molecules (N-CAMs) that appeared to be involved in two stages. These N-CAMs are involved first in induction of the neural plate, neural tube, notocord, and somites, and secondly in inductive events in neural crest cell development as well as in the ontogeny of various neural structures and other organs. In the induction, for example, of cardiac mesoderm and limb buds, the appearance of N-CAMs was highly dynamic and transient, whereas in the neural crest cells, N-CAMs appeared early, disappeared during migration, and reappeared at sites where ganglia were forming [53]. In the neural tube region, N-CAMs were present at all stages; N-CAMs were not found on glial cells. These findings led Edelman and colleagues to propose that adhesion during early embryogenesis and later histogenesis may be mediated by N-CAMs.

Differences in the carbohydrate structures of N-CAM were found between adult and embryonic brains in Edelman's laboratory [54]. The adult and embryonic forms of N-CAM differed in their mobilities on sodium dodecyl sulfate–polyacrylamide gel electrophoresis (SDS-PAGE). The embryonic form migrated in a broad region ranging in apparent molecular weight from 200,000 to 250,000, whereas the adult form migrated primarily in two bands of apparent molecular weights of 150,000 and 180,000.

The amino acid, amino sugar, and neutral sugar compositions of the embryonic and adult N-CAMs were similar. Limited amino- and carboxyl-terminal sequence analyses gave identical residues. Tryptic peptide maps of the two proteins were nearly identical, as were cyanogen bromide (CNBr) cleavage and limited proteolysis patterns. In striking contrast to these similarities, however, was the fact that the adult N-CAMs contained only 10% sialic acid as compared with 30% in embryonic N-CAMs. Further, after treatment of these molecules with neuraminidase, both embryonic and adult N-CAMs migrated on sodium dodecyl sulfate-polyacrylamide gel electrophoresis as a closely spaced doublet with an apparent molecular weight of 140,000, suggesting that the primary difference in the two forms of N-CAM is their sialic acid content. These findings led these workers [53,54] to put forward the hypothesis that postnatally, a transition in the carbohydrate portion of N-CAM occurs from the embryonic to the adult form. This raises the possibility that such a transition may act to stabilize neuronal patterns of adhesion in their final form.

Clearly, it would be anticipated that the presence of a teratogen that affects membrane fluidity and membrane structure might compromise the fundamental processes involved in synaptogenesis. It is well established that ethanol alters neuronal membrane fluidity. Recently, it has been shown that ethanol exposure during the brain growth spurt in the rat significantly decreases the sialic acid content of synaptosomes [55].

The fundamental processes essential to normal synaptogenesis, especially the development of growth cones and the recognition and adhesion processes, inevitably underlie any theory of brain ontogeny. The work of Edelman and associates (reviewed by Edelman [56]), indicates that the first of these primary processes likely to be understood is that of cell-cell adhesion. Cell-cell adhesion, cell-substrate adhesion, and intercellular junction adhesion appear to be mediated by completely different families of molecules. However, N-CAMs appear to be the most specific. Edelman [56] identified three distinct epochs of N-CAM function: inductive events in the formation of organ rudiments during early embryogenesis; events in neurohistogenesis (i.e., synaptogenetic events); and events occurring in the adult (i.e., possible neuronal cell surface regulation of cellular metabolic states).

Neuron-specific N-CAMs mediate neurite fasciculation, neuromuscular interaction, and orderly layering of neural tissue, while they undergo loss of sialic acid during development. A failure in the latter process is closely correlated with connectional disorders in the staggerer mutant in the mouse [57]. The available data on N-CAMs favor a modulation theory rather than a strict chemoaffinity theory of cellular recognition and adhesion [56]. Continued research in N-CAM chemistry promises to move toward the realization of a soundly based theory of molecular neuroontogeny.

5 SYNAPTIC GLYCOCONJUGATES AND RELATED SYNTHETIC AND METABOLIC ENZYMES

Contained within the presynaptic element are the presynaptic vesicles and presynaptic dense projections, and within the postsynaptic element are the postsynaptic densities. Pre- and postsynaptic paramembraneous densities consist of filamentous proteins. The synaptic cleft also contains proteinaceous, carbohydrate-rich material. The membranes of the presynaptic element have specific properties that permit vesicle-membrane interaction and initiation of the process of exocytosis. The neurotransmitter molecules thus released then interact with post- and/or presynaptic receptors in or on the synaptic membrane surfaces. It is thought that glycoconjugates are involved in many, if not all, of these synaptic events.

The chief chemical components of the neuronal plasma membrane implicated in neuronal ordering phenomena are the glycoconjugates. These components are anchored in the hydrophobic portion of the membrane and extend hydrophilic peptide and/or carbohydrate moieties into the intercellular space. The presence of glycosyltransferases [58] and carbohydrate-binding proteins (endogenous lectins) further emphasize the importance of glycosyltransferases in the recognition process.

It seems likely that synaptic membrane differentiation or specialization is the result of a change in the population of membrane glycoconjugates during the expansion of axon terminals and dendritic branches. The change in population of glycoconjugates may be brought about by the insertion of new glycoconjugates in the leading edge of the advancing growth cone. The resulting SPM has its own characteristic population of glycoconjugates, depending on the types of neurons constituting the particular synaptic connection. That is, each type of neuron has its own cell surface "signature" in the form of differing amounts of certain carbohydrate residues. This is controlled by the cell's genome and its synthetic machinery, which nevertheless are also subject to epigenetic influences, e.g. nutritional status, and the presence or absence of teratogens.

5.1 Synaptic Glycoproteins

Glycoproteins are thought to be involved in cell surface functions during synaptogenesis, especially in cell-cell recognition and in intracellular adhesion [40,59–61] and in the regulation of regional brain differentiation [39]. As pointed out by Brunngraber [62], glycoproteins are synthesized within the cell in order to subserve an extracellular function. Synapse-specific glycoproteins, proteins, and transmitter binding sites were identified in synaptic junctions by Mena et al. [63], who showed that concanavalin A-binding glycoproteins and kainic acid-binding sites are specific markers for synaptic junctions. In a later study, Mena and Cotman [64] isolated four glycoproteins of the rat synaptic junction by affinity chromatography. Tryptic peptide maps of these glycoproteins showed that the three largest glycoproteins contained a high percentage of identical peptides and that the amino acid sequences thereof have a high degree of homology. Their findings suggest that homologous glycoproteins participate in synapse formation and/or synapse maintenance. However, the mechanisms underlying glycoprotein participation in synapse formation are not clear.

The carbohydrate moieties of glycoproteins in neural tissue generally consist of fucose, N-acetylneuraminic acid, galactose, mannose, glucosamine, and galactosamine. Carbohydrate usually constitutes 60–80% of purified glycopeptides. According to Roseman [60], the oligosaccharide chains of both glycolipids and gangliosides are not synthesized by a template mechanism. Instead, the expression of the appropriate genes for the synthesis of each type of glycoprotein apparently produces, in each case, a complex of multiglycosyltransferases. The oligosaccharide chains are then built either by adding monosaccharides to the ends of growing oligosaccharide chains, or by the addition of di-, tri-, or even higher oligosaccharides.

After investigating the process of cellular adhesion, Roseman [60] concluded that each cell surface is covered by a mosaic of complex carbohydrates and glycosyltransferases, i.e. the cell surface contains both substrates and enzymes. Another conclusion was that the binding of substrate on one cell to enzyme on another cell results in adhesion of the two cells. This theory of adhesiveness also provides an explanation for the modification of intercellular adhesive strength.

Barondes [40] emphasized the role of glycoproteins during synaptogenesis because of their greater structural variability and the enormous volume occupied by their long, extensively hydrated polysaccharide chains, which extend far out from the membrane surface, a characteristic that would promote intercellular interaction. However, he also pointed out the importance of glycolipids in the process of cell recognition. Glycolipids are more concentrated in brain than in other organs and are particularly concentrated in nerve endings.

A major finding in Barondes's laboratory [40] was that there is extensive synthesis of glycoproteins during synaptogenesis in rodents. He pointed out the capacity of nerve terminals to add carbohydrate residues to polypeptides synthesized in the neuronal perikaryon as well as the synthesis of several high-molecular-weight glycoproteins during this stage of development. He also observed that the rate of synthesis of these compounds markedly diminished during days 10–15 after birth. In view of these data Barondes [40] proposed a model for interneuronal recognition during the establishment of synaptic connectivities based on the complementarity of cell surfaces, previously observed in the retinotectal system [65,66].

Brunngraber [59] has also stressed the role of glycoproteins. He held that during synaptogenesis the probing axon tip with its distinctive "code," consisting of a specific arrangement of sugar residues, will pass by inappropriate targets as it searches and finds its appropriate target. In his view, the individuality and stage of life of a cell is defined by its arrangement of the hexose-hexosamine matrix from which fucose and N-acetylneuraminic acid residues project.

During development in the rat the changes in synaptic sialoglycoproteins [67], changes in sialidase specificity [68], and developmentally related changes in biosynthetic labeling properties of sialic acid residues [69] suggest the existence of structurally distinct populations of sialooligosaccharides. These populations demonstrate different metabolic properties serving as substrates for sialidase at different developmental ages. Furthermore, as a result of their studies of developmental changes in glycoproteins in the developing chick nervous system, Mintz and colleagues [70] suggest that each particular region of the brain may show a unique glycoprotein pattern.

Developmentally related changes in the carbohydrate composition of synaptic glycoproteins were described by Federico and DiBenedetta [71]. According to these authors, the developmental patterns of glycopeptides and glycoproteins are very similar in humans and rats. They also pointed out that the sialic acid in the insoluble glycoproteins resembles closely that of gangliosides. Van Den Eijnden and colleagues reported that the sialoglycoprotein level in rats appeared to increase twofold from birth to 20 days of age [72]. This correlates with the outgrowth of neuronal processes over the same time period. However, they found that both the synthetase and transferase enzyme activities were highest at birth and tended to decrease during maturation. They interpreted this to mean that at some stages in early neonatal development, sialyltransferase is present in structures other than synaptic membranes, since the newborn rat brain is nearly devoid of synapses. They found that the developmental profile of endogenous sialic acid accepting molecules was very similar to that of sialoglycoproteins. From this they concluded that sialoglycoprotein synthesis during postnatal development is not limited by synthetase and transferase activities alone, but may depend largely on the production of endogenous sialoglycoprotein acceptors, which may be precursors of sialoglycoproteins.

Glycoproteins are also present in synaptic cleft material. Mena and Cotman [64] found that homologous glycoproteins may participate in synapse formation or maintenance or both. They suggest that one type of glycoprotein may be associated with a particular class of synapses, or that the glycoproteins may have different functions at the same synapse.

5.2 Synaptic Glycolipids (Gangliosides)

In the adult mammalian brain, from rodent to primate, ganglioside concentrations and patterns are similar, and similar changes in ganglioside concentration and pattern occur during development [73]. Gangliosides are abundant and very active metabolically in synapses, whereas in myelin the ganglioside level is low and the metabolic activity is greatly reduced [74].

The high concentration and uniformity of composition of gangliosides in the nervous system suggest that gangliosides serve a special purpose in nerve tissue [75]. They are enriched at the synaptic junction, where they bind calcium ions with high affinity. Thus Svennerholm [75] proposed that the role of gangliosides at the synaptic junction is to bind the calcium ions released at each impulse and transported via specific channels into the presynaptic terminal. The removal of calcium ions from gangliosides leads to instability of the presynaptic membrane and facilitates fusion of presynaptic vesicles with the membrane. The increased calcium ion concentration within the presynaptic terminal results in contraction of the microfilaments and subsequent ejection of transmitter molecules, i.e. exocytosis. Further, Svennerholm [75] suggests that gangliosides may also participate in reuptake of neurotransmitter molecules into the presynaptic terminal.

Hess et al [76] hypothesized that if gangliosides are highly localized in neuronal surface membranes and synapses, they should be particularly concentrated in grey matter regions of the brain, e.g. in the frontal association cortex of the human, or in rat somatosensory cortex. If so, the assay of ganglioside sialic acid should provide an index of the absolute and relative mass of axon and dendritic processes and their synaptic connections together with the glial membranes that compartmentalize these structures. Unfortunately, light and electron microscope techniques for the quantitation of neuronal membrane and synaptic parameters are excessively laborious and often inaccurate. However, a combination of quantitative histochemical assays with cell counting should prove useful in assessing the neuronal basis of neurological function. The ganglioside sialic acid content, expressed per neuron or per cell, is an abstraction, as was pointed out by Bass [77]. It is an average for all of the neurons, or cells, in the region under study. Also, the number of synapses per neuron varies with type of neuron and is not related to size of neuron. However, all variables considered, the assay of sialic acid may be the most convenient and accurate method for detecting quantitative differences between normal and abnormal brains. The studies of Bass [77] support the validity and usefulness of estimations of ganglioside sialic acid content per cell or per neuron as an index of the relative mass of neuronal plasma membranes and their derivatives in neural tissues.

Bass [77], Hess and Pope [78], and Hess et al. [76] found similar quantities of ganglioside sialic acid, expressed per unit dry weight, in human frontal cortex and rat somatosensory cortex. Their combined microchemical assays and cytoarchitectonic studies revealed that the distribution of sialogangliosides in the layers of frontal human cortex and rat somatosensory cortex paralleled the occurrence of high concentrations of dendritic and axonal plexuses and synaptic connections. The total ganglioside sialic acid content, expressed per cell or neuron, in human frontal cortex greatly exceeded that of rat somatosensory cortex. According to a number of workers [79,80] increases in ganglioside sialic acid accurately reflect axodendritic proliferation during peak synaptogenesis. This supports the hypothesis of Bass [77] that ganglioside sialic acid can serve as a quantitative index of synaptic integrity in cognitive disorders of development and aging.

5.3 Glycosyltransferases and Sialyltransferases

The synthesis and integration of glycoconjugates into SPMs is of importance in understanding the composition and function of these membranes. Dreyfus et al. [81] studied sialyltransferase activity in two neuronal models, retina and cultures of isolated neurons. They determined that part of the activity in pure neuronal cells is located on the external surface of the neuronal plasma membranes. These findings support the hypothesis of Roseman [60] that ectoglycosyltransferases are implicated in cellular recognition and adhesion processes. Dreyfus et al. [81] assumed that the gangliosides located on the neuronal membrane surface were derived in part from synthesis by the Golgi apparatus and in part by synthesis at their location on the membrane surface. More information is needed in order to determine whether these ectoenzyme systems act on glycoprotein substrates. In either case, glycolipids or glycoproteins, several transferases are needed. Some of the specific enzymatic steps, as reported by Dreyfus et al [81], were similar in the two-model systems studied.

Ng and Dain [82] were able to distinguish between glycolipid sialyltransferase activities and glycoprotein sialyltransferase activities. Typically, both of these enzyme systems are membrane-bound. The developmental patterns of these two systems have been shown to be distinctly different [83].

The activities of glycoprotein sialyltransferase decline dramatically during early development [72]. In another study reported by Van Den Eijnden and Van Dijk [84], it was concluded that glycoprotein sialyltransferase in the adult brain of the rat and calf are localized, at least for the greater part, in neuronal membranes other than synaptic complexes. These authors stated that they had previously found that sialyltransferases were present also on membranes of glial cells occurring in both grey and white matter.

Preti et al. [85] found an enrichment of sialyltransferase activity in the synaptosomal membrane fraction as well as activity in the subcellular fractions. They also found that the synaptosomal membranes carried at least two different sialyltransferase activities, one acting on lactosylceramide and glycolipid acceptors and the other acting on DS-fetuin and glycoprotein acceptors. Additional studies of these enzyme systems and their possible role in neuronal cell recognition and adhesion are needed.

During the past decade the methodology for the analysis of carbohydrates in glycoproteins and glycolipids has become reliable and is now capable of supplying the absolute composition, sequence, and configuration of the carbohydrate residues [86]. The presence of carbohydrate moieties in many glycoproteins has been found to be essential in providing functionality to, and in preserving structural integrity of, the molecule. Thus, if exposure of the developing brain to a specific teratogen affects the carbohydrate moieties of glycoproteins and/or glycolipids, the structural integrity and subsequently the function of the membrane is likely to be affected.

6 AN ANIMAL MODEL OF THE HUMAN BRAIN GROWTH SPURT

6.1 Timing of the Brain Growth Spurt Relative to Birth

The brain growth spurt in the rat is completely postnatal, whereas in the human it is perinatal. According to some reports, the neuroontogenetic events occurring during postnatal days 4–7 in the rat are closely comparable to those occurring during the third trimester in the human [87–89]. Samson and Diaz [87] state that for comparable exposure during the prenatal portion of the brain growth spurt in the human, the rat must be exposed through postnatal day 8. However, Adlard et al. [90] had previously proposed that the rat brain at postnatal day 5 has reached a stage of development comparable with the human infant at term.

In an analytical review of brain growth stages, Gottlieb et al. [22] suggested that there are three discrete phases of rapid growth during the brain growth spurt in the rodent brain, i.e., during postnatal days 0–6, 8–12, and 17–23. They noted two growth plateaus or slow-growth phases during days 6–8 and 12–17. The information presented by these authors, summarized from a critical review of a number of published studies, suggests that the most rapid rate of growth in the rodent brain occurs during postnatal days 8–12, the peak of the entire brain growth spurt in the rat occurring at about the midpoint of this time period. Thus, in the rat brain peak growth rate occurs on about day 9 or 10 after birth [22], whereas the peak rate of the human brain growth spurt occurs just prior to birth [25]. Therefore, it is likely that rat brain development during postnatal days 4–10 is most closely comparable to that occurring in the human brain during the prenatal portion of its brain growth spurt.

According to Dobbing and Smart [27], about one-eighth of the critically vulnerable brain growth spurt occurs before birth in the human. The various studies discussed above suggest that a comparable portion of the brain growth spurt in the rat is completed at least by postnatal day 10. In these terms, the postnatal rat is a suitable animal model for investigations of the effects of ethanol and/or various other agents during the brain growth spurt. Studies conducted during this time period in an animal model are relevant to the developing human brain. Therefore, if ethanol exposure during the brain growth spurt in the rat leads to permanent central nervous system damage, the potential danger from exposure of the fetal human brain to ethanol during the third trimester should be taken seriously.

Because of the rapid rate of dendritic and axonal membrane elaboration during synaptogenesis, the synapse may be a prime target of ethanol during the brain growth spurt. If the extremely sensitive or susceptible dendritic and axonal growth cones are exposed to ethanol at this time, the membrane-fluidizing effects of ethanol may interfere with fundamental processes underlying the development of specificity in the molecular structure of the outer surface of the membrane, the initiation of formation of the growth cone, and the movement of the leading edge of the growth cone toward and its recognition of dendritic target sites. Also, altered synaptic membrane molecular structure as well as altered membrane fluidity may affect the adhesive mechanisms essential to the establishment of synaptic connections.

6.2 Interspecies Similarities and Differences

The general sequence of neuroontogenetic events shows no species differences [91], and the anatomical units (neurons, glia, endothelial cells) differ little from one species to another. Myelin shows only minor species differences. Rat neurons have composition and electrical properties similar to those in the human and show numerous similar drug responses. Nevertheless, in spite of this wealth of similarities, there exist—as Dobbing [91] points out—two important species differences. These are the final complexities of the brain, and the timing of the brain growth spurt with respect to birth.

6.3 Subtle Damaging Effects of Ethanol on Synapses

Even though ethanol exposure during the brain growth spurt may be relatively brief in duration and/or relatively low in intensity, synaptic structures may be damaged during this period of increased susceptibility. Because of the large number of synaptic structures and their extensive distribution throughout brain tissue, the resulting damage is likely to be widespread and subtle. It may even be that the resulting damage will not be detectable at either the light or electron microscope level. However, if this is the case, it may be demonstrable at the membrane molecular level by various biochemical or cytohistochemical studies. Although subtle, alterations in synaptic membrane molecular structure may have serious consequences for brain function. These alterations may interfere with presynaptic mechanisms involved in neurotransmitter synthesis, storage, release, and uptake, as well as with postsynaptic mechanisms mediating neurotransmitter-receptor interactions and neurotransmitter disposition, or with both pre- and postsynaptic receptor properties. The damaging effects of ethanol during synaptogenesis may be reflected at all levels of biological organization, from the molecular to the behavioral and social, because the integrity of both synaptic structure and function are key factors subserving perception, arousal, cognition, emotion, motivation, reinforcement, and motor control—all of which are among the determinants of behavior.

6.4 Critical Intensity, Duration, and Timing of Ethanol Exposure

The intensity of the ethanol exposure at or above which subtle molecular damage to synaptic structures may result during synaptogenesis is not known. The duration of ethanol exposures of differing intensities that may cause synaptic molecular pathology during this time is also not known. Nor is it clear whether the resulting damage is due to the peak height of the blood ethanol concentration (BEC), to the total dosage of ethanol, or to both. Within the brain growth spurt in rodents, there are peak and plateau phases of growth rate [22]. Whether corresponding phases of the growth rate occur in the human brain growth spurt is not known. If so, it is likely that the susceptibility of the brain to damage varies with the peak and plateau growth rates. Because of the extreme vulnerability of rapidly growing tissues, if there is ever a time during brain ontogeny when relatively low BECs and/or short durations of ethanol exposure are capable of causing damage to developing synapses it is likely to be during the brain growth spurt.

7 METHODS OF ADMINISTRATION OF ETHANOL IN NEONATAL ANIMALS

7.1 Methodological Difficulties

Numerous methodological difficulties have hampered studies of the effects of ethanol in neonatal animals. Currently used methods include administration of ethanol 1) in liquid diet to the dam and via the dam's milk to neonates; 2) via inhalation to the dam and neonates simultaneously during the treatment period (9 h hours on one or two days) or to neonates while separated temporarily from dams (90 min per treatment twice daily); 3) via chronic gastric gavage with neonates isolated from dams throughout the period of treatment (4 days); and, 4) via intermittent gastric gavage with neonates separated from dams briefly (about 5 min per treatment of entire litter).

7.2 Ethanol Administration via the Dam's Milk

Ethanol administered via the dam's milk [92–96] affects neonates but also affects maternal nutritional status [97], milk production and ejection [98], and maternal behavior. All of these maternal effects indirectly affect neonates, thus confounding interpretation of results.

7.3 Ethanol Administration via Inhalation

Ethanol administered via inhalation to dams with their litters [99], or to neonates separated temporarily from dams [100], allows entry of ethanol vapors directly into arterial blood without prior passage through the liver. Ethanol vapors irritate respiratory epithelium and may lead to systemic metabolic changes. The high BEC in pups and their dams for long periods of time (9h of exposure plus the time required for disappearance of ethanol from the animals' bloodstream), or in pups upon their return to dams immediately after treatment, may affect pup-maternal interactions. Again, these factors confound interpretation of results.

7.4 Ethanol Administration in Artificially Reared Neonates

During the past few years, artificial rearing of neonatal rats independently of dams with ethanol administered via surgically implanted intragastric tubes [101–104] has resulted in microcephaly and other FAS-like characteristics. Problems associated with this method include high mortality [105], a 12.5% lower body weight in experimental animals than in pups reared by dams [106], questionable effects of anesthetic and surgical procedures, surgical infections (e.g., peritonitis), retardation of gastric emptying [107], and the separation of pups from dams and littermates throughout the entire treatment period. Rearing pups in isolation is known to affect the cerebral cortex and the hippocampus [108,109]. Differential rearing affects synaptogenesis, dendritic branching, subsynaptic plates, and synaptic curvature [110–112]. Any of these factors is likely to confound the results.

7.5 Fractional Dosage of Ethanol via Gastric Gavage

If the objective is to mimic in an animal model the intensity and duration of ethanol exposure associated with moderate to heavy social drinking in the human rather than that associated with alcoholism *per se*, then fractional dosage via gastric gavage can be used. Gastric gavage enables study of the direct effects of ethanol, allows administration of exact amounts of ethanol to each neonate, and facilitates sampling for BEC at designated time intervals after treatment. It enables the attainment of desired BECs (e.g., ethanol 4 g/kg at the age studied results in BECs in range 234–304 mg/dl, at the peak of the ethanol disappearance curve [55,113,117]. Further, an entire litter is separated from the dam only for about 5 min per treatment. Retrieval of pups by dams is not significantly affected. Pups spontaneously attach to dams' nipples within about 10 min following treatment. The effects of ethanol on body weight associated with this method are minimal, as observed at the end of an 11-day treatment period, and catchup, with respect to this parameter, is complete by 70 days of age [113]. The mortality in ethanol-treated and sham-treated controls, using fractional doses via gastric gavage, was not found to differ in these studies.

8 RECENT ETHANOL STUDIES IN NEONATAL ANIMALS

Many investigators have examined the effects of ethanol exposure in animals during gestation. Some have expanded the experimental period to include both gestation and lactation. Relatively few studies have been focused exclusively on the early postnatal period. However, the mammalian central nervous system has been shown to be vulnerable to ethanol during early postnatal life, particularly during the brain growth spurt [55,87,100,101,103–105,114–119].

Ethanol exposure of the developing brain during lactation by the administration of ethanol to the dam and then via the dam's milk to preweanling rat pups resulted in higher mortality and retarded growth [94], lower levels of DNA and RNA [92], increased seizure activity [120], decreased aggressive behavior [95]; altered emotional reactivity [93], and learning deficits [96].

Ethanol exposure of preweanling rats via inhalation [100,114], on postnatal days 3 and 4 only resulted in a mean BEC of 268 mg/dl and caused a significant permanent reduction in the number of Purkinje cells in all cerebellar lobules, with no further reduction upon exposure throughout postnatal days 3–20. Brain weight was significantly reduced (20%) in the ethanol-treated animals. Ethanol exposure of preweanling rats and their dams via inhalation for 9 h on either day 3 or days 3 and 4 after birth resulted in BECs in the range of 552–562 mg/dl [99]. Purkinje cells, on day 5 after birth, were reduced in number in lobe I by approximately 47% and decreased in density in lobe VIII by approximately 45%. Cerebellar weight was reduced by 4%. The mean BEC value in this study by Phillips and Cragg [99] was approximately two times greater than that in the study performed by Bauer-Moffett and Altman [100]. Whether the animals treated by Phillips and Cragg [99] would have survived for testing in early adulthood is not known, since apparently all of the animals exposed to ethanol were used in studies performed on day 5 after birth.

In an ultrastructural study Jones and Colangelo [118,119] examined three groups of rats (control, ethanol-treated, and ethanol-rehabilitated) at various ages between 7 and 76 postnatal days. Ethanol vapor administration (BEL 0.1 g/100 ml) was commenced at 3 postnatal days. Ultrastructural differences in the neocortical synapses analyzed were only evident at 56 and 76 days, perforated synapses being most common in the 56-day ethanol-treated material and degenerating synapses in the 56-day ethanol-rehabilitated material. The authors considered that at 56 days synaptic remodeling is under way in the ethanol-treated material, whereas following rehabilitation the terminals are relatively immature and appear to be actively functioning.

Studies of preweanling rats reared independently of the dam [106,107] with ethanol included in the diet [87,89,101–105] have revealed significantly increased mortality. Sham-operated groups also showed increased mortality. The ethanol treated groups showed significant reductions (19–20%) in brain weight, microcephaly, and FAS-like brain and behavioral deficits. Sex differences relative to the severity of the effects of ethanol during early postnatal life have also been reported [105]. A study of the effects of ethanol exposure during days postnatal 1–10 in rats artificially reared [104] revealed dramatic alterations in the hippocampal mossy fiber organization and aberrant intra- and infrapyramidal mossy fiber projections to CA3a and CA3b. The distribution of the infrapyramidal mossy fiber field was reduced in pair-fed controls, reared in isolation, as compared with animals reared with their dams. An increased distribution of the mossy fiber fields was observed in the ethanol-exposed animals compared with pair-fed controls. West et al. [104] pointed out that exposure to ethanol during the equivalent of the third trimester may be more deleterious to brain development than exposure during the first two trimesters.

Problems associated with the administration of ethanol to preweanling animals (via either the dam's milk or inhalation, or by artificial rearing combined with chronic gastric intubation) discourage use of these methods. Fractional dosage of ethanol via gastric gavage, as recommended by Sonderegger and colleagues [121] and Burns and colleagues [55,117], avoids the disadvantages of previously used methods and offers several advantages (Section 7.5).

9 MEMBRANE EFFECTS OF ETHANOL IN NEONATAL ANIMALS

Klemm and colleagues [122–125] have shown that sialic acid is a useful biochemical marker for the effects of ethanol on neuronal membranes. Sialic acid, a terminal carbohydrate residue of oligosaccharide and polysaccharide chains of glycolipids and glycoproteins, is an integral part of the neuronal membrane. It is located on the surface of the membrane and extends into the extracellular space [126]. In addition to its role in cellular recognition and adhesion, it modulates sodium and calcium binding [127], causes electronegativity of cell surfaces [128], is a component of several receptors [129], and is necessary for neurotransmission [127,130]. Sialic acid is more concentrated in synaptosomes than in brain homogenates [62].

Ethanol 4 g/kg body weight daily administered in two fractional doses 3 h apart via gastric intubation throughout the brain growth spurt (postnatal days 6–16) in rats resulted in significantly reduced sialic acid concentration in synaptosomes with an equally distributed decrease of glycoprotein-bound and glycolipid-bound sialic acid; a significantly diminished activity of ectosialyltransferase with asialofetuin as exogenous acceptor; no change in neuraminidase activity; and no change in either total protein or lipid [55]. These findings indicate that the reduction of synaptosomal sialic acid by ethanol exposure during the brain growth spurt is caused, at least in part, by an inhibition of the incorporation of sialic acid into synaptosomal membrane-bound sialoglycomacromolecules by ectosialyltransferase. In a recent study using the same animal model [131], a significant increase in synaptosomal galactose was found. Further studies should be done to show whether ethanol exposure during this phase of neuroontogeny may also inhibit the intracellular biosynthesis of sialoglycomacromolecules, e.g. in the Golgi apparatus, where primary synthesis of glycoconjugates is considered to occur. The resulting altered molecular structure of synaptic surface membranes is likely to affect synaptic function and might be reflected in developmental cognitive disorders.

Micromorphological studies performed on littermates of animals used for the above synaptosomal studies revealed nonsignificant structural changes in the cerebellum, lobule IX, at the light and electron microscope levels [117]. It may be that subtle damage, detectable by biochemical means, is not being detected by conventional morphological studies. Synaptic biochemical molecular changes, however, are likely to be reflected in altered synaptic function and thus may have serious consequences.

In another study on the same animal model [132], no effect on body temperature was found in response to ethanol at the times tested (on the 1st, 4th, 7th,and 11th days of treatment). The absence of a hypothermic response on these test days during the 11 consecutive days of treatment does not suggest that tolerance to ethanol has developed. The poikilothermic rat may not be capable of developing tolerance at the age of treatment in response to the dosage used and the relatively short duration of ethanol exposure (approximately 8–9 h per day rather than continuously for 24 h per day). Littleton [133] states that it is practically impossible for weanling mice to develop central nervous system tolerance to ethanol. However, Hitzemann and Harris [50] found no significant age-dependent effect of ethanol on membrane fluidity; rather, their data suggested that membrane organization subserving ethanol sensitivity is present and operative by day 3 after birth. Majchrowicz and Hunt [134] suggested that the length of time necessary for tolerance to develop is dependent upon the total amount consumed per day. With the low-dosage level (4 g/kg body weight), it is not surprising that a hypothermic response was not observed in these animals.

No changes were observed in synaptosomal ATPase activity in preweanling animals treated with ethanol throughout the brain growth spurt [131], which further suggests that tolerance had not developed. Also, no alterations were found in either cholesterol or phospholipid content (unpublished observation) in synaptosomal preparations from ethanol-treated as compared with control groups. It has been suggested that the development of tolerance to ethanol is dependent on an increase in the cholesterol content of neuronal membranes [52].

Other findings in studies using this animal model include permanently decreased brain weights (with no difference in body weights), disproportionately and permanently reduced cerebellar weights, a significantly diminished number of cerebellar cells, and altered balancing ability [113].

In additional animals, the dose of ethanol was increased to 6 g/kg administered via gastric gavage in two fractional dosages, 3 h apart, on one day only (postnatal day 6). The effects of this dose of ethanol administered on one day only also significantly and permanently affected whole-brain and cerebellar weights and the number of cerebellar cells, without affecting body weight [113]. These findings with relatively low dosages of ethanol (4 and 6 g/kg are approximately one-third and one-half, respectively, of doses often used in preweanling rats) reflect the crucially vulnerable status of the brain during the brain growth spurt. The recent report of a significantly lower birth weight in the human following maternal intake of one or two drinks per day [135] further emphasizes the potential dangers of low levels of ethanol exposure during development.

10 ETHANOL TOLERANCE/DEPENDENCE

Elucidation of the biochemical and biophysical correlates of intoxication, tolerance, and addiction is important to the control and prevention of alcohol abuse and alcoholism. Knowledge of the mechanisms underlying these effects of ethanol in mature organisms should promote better understanding of the teratogenic effects of ethanol on the developing brain.

10.1 Changes Induced in the Brain by Ethanol

It is known that the administration of a single dose of ethanol results in nonspecific general depression of the CNS and subsequent behavioral changes, the severity of which is dose-dependent or BEC-dependent [136]. Upon clearance of ethanol from the blood, the CNS returns to a relatively normal state. However, hangover effects suggest longer-lasting CNS changes, which even now are poorly understood. Long-term drinking induces longer-lasting changes in the brain. Upon termination of long-term drinking, and elimination of ethanol from the system, the ethanol withdrawal syndrome appears. Ethanol withdrawal consists of a state of hyperexcitability that represents a reversal of the depressed state during intoxication.

10.2 Dependency and Withdrawal

The natural history of ethanol dependency in the human or in the experimental animal, as described by Majchrowicz [136], includes the predrinking period, the drinking period (pharmacologically defined as the induction period), and the alcohol withdrawal period. These three periods reflect three different functional states of the CNS. The predrinking period reflects a normal CNS functional state and serves as a reference or control state. During the drinking period the CNS is nonspecifically depressed by the high BEC. Upon discontinuance of drinking, the ethanol withdrawal syndrome appears. In the first phase of withdrawal there is essentially a continuation of CNS depression that gradually lessens to a somewhat normal state. In the second phase of withdrawal, physical dependence is overtly expressed in signs and reactions reflecting the hyperexcitability of the CNS. Dependency is not manifested until the BEC declines to or below a threshold level. After recovery from withdrawal the brain may eventually return to the predrinking state.

10.3 The Possible Role of Acetaldehyde

Majchrowicz and Hunt [137] addressed the issues of the possible role of acetaldehyde in intoxication and dependence and the inhibitory effects of acetaldehyde and ethanol on brain metabolism. Based on the ratio of the 50% lethal dose (LD_{50}) of ethanol to that of acetaldehyde under *in vivo* conditions, the role of acetaldehyde in the actions of ethanol has yet to be established. They pointed out that various studies have shown that the effects of acetaldehyde (very low in the blood of intoxicated chronic alcoholics) and ethanol exert only low-grade effects on brain metabolism. They also pointed out that the effects of ethanol upon the brain relate more to the neuronal membrane than to changes in neuronal metabolism.

Blakley and Scott [138] determined that ethanol, not acetaldehyde, is the proximate teratogen of FAS in the mouse. Ethanol and acetaldehyde were administered independently to groups of pregnant CD mice, a strain known to be sensitive to ethanol teratogenesis. Coadministration of 4-methylpyrazol, a potent inhibitor of alcohol dehydrogenase, dramatically increased the embryotoxicity of ethanol, whereas coadministration of acetaldehyde did not affect embryotoxicity.

11 MEMBRANE EFFECTS OF ETHANOL

Ethanol is thought to cause its pharmacological effects by acting on neuronal membranes, particularly synaptic membranes. Although the molecular mechanisms underlying intoxication, tolerance, and dependence are not completely understood, evidence is accumulating that ethanol-induced fluidization of membranes is an important event in the development of tolerance. Tolerance has been defined as the consequence of a rapid adaptation of the synaptic membrane to the effects of long-term ethanol exposure [139], and that dependence occurs only when tolerance has reached a stage of irreversibility. It appears that the length of time necessary for physical dependence to be expressed as a withdrawal syndrome in rats depends on the total amount of ethanol consumed per day [134]. However, additional studies are needed to determine whether the withdrawal syndrome can follow lower total dosages that are given over a shorter duration of time which nevertheless can result in higher peak BECs.

11.1 Alterations of Membrane Fluidity

Chin and Goldstein showed that ethanol *in vitro* increased the fluidity of spin-labeled erythrocyte membranes [140] and also of brain membranes [141]. Further, they showed [141] that chronic *in vivo* exposure to ethanol attenuated the ethanol-induced fluidization of synaptosomal membranes. Goldstein and Chin [142] concluded that ethanol disorders membranes by disrupting the orderly packing between adjacent acyl chains, thus increasing the mobility of spin labels or fluorescent dyes in the membranes and shifting the phase transition to lower temperatures. This could affect protein function. Goldstein and Chin [142] previously found that the molar ratio of cholesterol to phospholipid increased from 0.706 to 0.739 in synaptosomal membranes of tolerant mice. As defined by Goldstein [143], membrane fluidity means a combination of different types of mobility of membrane components, including the flexibility of acyl chains, lateral diffusion of molecules within the plane of the membrane, transverse diffusion of molecules from one monolayer to another, and phase transitions leading to lateral phase separations. Ethanol may affect any of these factors. Goldstein et al. [144] found approximately a twofold increase in neuronal surface glycoconjugates in mice treated chronically with ethanol. They suggest that this change may be related to the effects of ethanol on the fluidity of neuronal membranes.

11.2 Alterations in Membrane Lipids

Johnson et al. [52] demonstrated that changes in lipid composition in synaptic membranes accounts at least in part for adaptation to ethanol-induced membrane fluidization. They removed cholesterol and trace nonpolar lipids from lipid extracts of tolerant and control mice. At this time it was not possible to detect any difference between tolerant and control membranes. They replaced cholesterol to provide a cholesterol-to-phospholipid ratio of 0.54 (the control group level) and were able to measure differences between tolerant and control lipid extracts. Thus, in addition to the influence of increased cholesterol, altered lipid composition was shown to play a role in the adaptation of membranes to long-term ethanol. Johnson et al. [145] observed apparent tolerance to the fluidizing effects of ethanol in both mice and rats. Acute *in vivo* ethanol exposure did not alter the ethanol-induced fluidity of the reconstituted membranes. Logan et al. [146] confirmed the observation that ethanol causes an increase in the fluidity of the lipid regions of the membrane.

Crews et al. [147] found a significantly increased cholesterol-to-phospholipid molar ratio in SPMs from dependent-intoxicated rats and a lesser increase in the molar ratio in rats undergoing withdrawal. In ethanol-dependent mice, significant increases in cholesterol content and in the cholesterol-to-phospholipid ratio were observed only in synaptosomal membranes [148]. The fatty acid content of SPM phospholipids did not differ significantly in any of the groups. A drastic decrease had been observed in phosphorus-labeled phosphatidylinosotol and phosphatidylserine in microsomes from rats during withdrawal [149]. There is also evidence that ethanol selectively decreases the unsaturated acyl groups of phosphatidylserine without altering the acyl composition of other phospholipids or sphingolipids [150]. However, chronic ethanol exposure in guinea pigs has been found to cause a 50% increase in SPM phosphatidylserine [151]. In another study Harris et al. [150] found that gangliosides enhance the membrane actions of ethanol, whereas Rubin and Rottenberg [152] have pointed out that the increased membrane rigidity resulting from chronic ethanol exposure makes SPMs resistant to disordering by ethanol.

11.3 Alterations of Calcium Transport

The work of Harris and Shroeder [153] suggests that the increases in the fluidity of membranes by low concentrations of ethanol are sufficient to interfere with ion transport. Harris and Hood [154] showed that ethanol inhibits depolarization-dependent calcium ion uptake in synaptosomes without affecting uptake under nondepolarizing conditions. Harris and Fenner [155] found increased intrasynaptosomal binding of calcium. This could modulate synaptic activity in two ways: first, by a reduction of the intrasynaptosomal levels of free calcium with subsequent alteration of calcium-dependent enzymes leading to a reduction of neurotransmitter release; second, by increased binding of calcium to the cytoplasmic membrane surface of the SPM, thereby affecting the physicochemical properties of this leaflet of the membrane. This would probably affect events in synaptic neurotransmission. Stokes and Harris [156] observed that ethanol *in vitro* inhibited potassium-, glutamate-, and veratridine-stimulated calcium uptake in synaptosomes. Further, they noted that cerebellar calcium channels are more sensitive than cerebral calcium channels to ethanol, and that cerebral sodium channels are more sensitive than cerebellar sodium channels to ethanol. A biphasic effect of ethanol on mitochondrial uptake of calcium was reported by Burke et al. [157], with enhanced uptake at low concentrations and inhibited uptake at high concentrations. This would also have an effect on synaptic function. There is additional evidence that the sodium ion gradient-dependent calcium uptake is very sensitive to ethanol [158].

11.4 Alterations in Membrane-Bound Enzymes

Ethanol in high concentrations disrupts neuronal membrane structure, particularly SPM structure. For example, ethanol in high doses increases the cholesterol-to-phospholipid ratio and affects orderly packing between adjacent acyl chains. Ethanol-induced alterations of neuronal membrane lipid constituents would be likely to affect the conformation of membrane-bound proteins residing in the membranes. Guerri and Grisolia [159] found that SPM-bound enzymes from ethanol-treated animals were more stable than those from controls. This evidence suggests a protein conformation change.

11.4.1 Alterations in adenylate cyclase. Adenylate cyclase, a membrane-bound protein residing on the inner leaflet of neuronal membranes, is activated by ethanol. However, the mechanism underlying its activation is unclear. The work of Rabin and Molinoff [160] indicates that there are multiple sites of action of ethanol on adenylate cyclase. Luthin and Tabakoff [161] found that ethanol does not affect the ability of calcium to activate adenylate cyclase. However, they observed that ethanol concentrations in the range of 50–75 mM (comparable to BECs found in their treated mice) altered adenylate cyclase activity in the presence of guanine nucleotides. Significant activation of adenylate cyclase by ethanol in concentrations less than 500 mM was not observed, except in the presence of guanine nucleotides, e.g. 5′-guanylylimidodiphosphate.

11.4.2 Alterations in Na^+/K^+-activated ATPase. Israel et al. [162] hypothesized that a compensatory increase in Na^+/K^+ ATPase activity may be responsible for tolerance of or physical dependence on ethanol, which might affect the enzyme either directly by interacting with the enzyme protein or indirectly by perturbing the membrane wherein it resides. Ethanol in high dosages is known to produce neuronal membrane disorganization [163]. Levental and Tabakoff [164] assessed the effects of chronic ethanol in mice on Na^+/K^+ ATPase activity, using a feeding regimen known to produce tolerance and dependence. They observed that Na^+/K^+-activated ATPase of mouse synaptosomal membranes is inhibited by high concentrations of ethanol. However, the enzyme from ethanol-tolerant mice was resistant to the inhibitory effects of ethanol and also had a lower transition temperature than that from controls. They suggested that resistance to the effects of ethanol on Na^+/K^+ ATPase might be related to ethanol tolerance.

In a review of the effects of ethanol on Na^+/K^+ ATPase, Roach [165] concluded that, although most studies had neither confirmed nor denied an *in vivo* effect of ethanol on brain synaptosomal Na^+/K^+ ATPase, this enzyme is inhibited by ethanol *in vitro* if the potassium ion concentration is sufficiently low. She pointed out that inhibition of the enzyme results from a lipophilic interaction of ethanol with the plasma membrane and requires at least 0.22 M ethanol for 50% inhibition. She suggests that it is unlikely that ethanol concentrations occurring *in vivo* during moderately severe intoxication (0.02–0.04 M) would be sufficient to suppress the enzyme significantly. In view of the correspondence between lipophilicity and pharmacological potency of lower aliphatic alcohols and other CNS depressants, it is likely that other membrane components more sensitive to hydrophobic modification than Na^+/K^+ ATPase may be responsible for the depressant action of these agents. If the enzyme is not inhibited *in vivo* by ethanol, then the hypothesis that the enzyme activity increases during chronic ethanol intake as an adaptative response to counteract its inhibition by ethanol is not supported. The increased activity of the enzyme in the CNS seems to be related to the hyperexcitability associated with withdrawal. According to Roach [165], the changes that result in greater activity of the enzyme may be an increased net synthesis of the protein components of the enzyme complex, activation of the enzyme by altered membrane conformation, or a change in the available activators or inhibitors of the enzyme.

Beauge et al. [166] observed synaptosomal membrane disordering related to acute ethanol administration in naive and short-term ethanol-intoxicated rats. They found no change in basal intrinsic membrane fluidity as measured by fluorescence polarization. Na^{+}/K^{+} ATPase activity was found to be increased slightly in both experimental groups. Following addition of ethanol *in vitro*, fluidizing and Na^{+}/K^{+} ATPase-inhibiting effects were markedly increased 18 h after administration of ethanol (5 g/kg body weight via gastric gavage) to naive rats. The hypersensitization was no longer apparent in short-term intoxicated rats (pretreated for 4 days). The disappearance of hypersensitivity may reflect an early stage of tolerance development.

Fleuret-Balter et al. [167] pointed out that basal values of membrane parameters are poor indicators of ethanol action, membrane fluidity, and Na^{+}/K^{+} ATPase activity. Therefore, their focus was on *in vitro* ethanol-induced sensitivity. As in their previous study [166] they examined both membrane fluidity and Na^{+}/K^{+} ATPase activity. *In vitro* ethanol produced an increased membrane fluidity and an inhibition of enzyme activity in a concentration-dependent manner in synaptosomes from acute and short-term ethanol-treated and control animals. After a single dose of ethanol in a naive animal the sensitivity to ethanol added *in vitro* was enhanced, as revealed both by changes in membrane fluidity and Na^{+}/K^{+} ATPase activity. The significant increase in basal Na^{+}/K^{+} ATPase activity *in vitro* without any change in basal membrane fluidity suggests that the change in enzyme activity may not be due to a modification of the lipid environment. Further studies are needed to determine the mechanism of the membrane hypersensitivity after acute ethanol exposure in a naive animal.

Later studies by Beauge et al. [168] suggest that synaptosomal Na^{+}/K^{+} ATPase activity may serve as an index of tolerance to ethanol. They determined the activity of the enzyme, its sensitivity to ethanol added *in vitro*, and the interaction of norepinephrine-ethanol with the enzyme *in vitro* during the development of tolerance in the rat. In their treatment regimen, functional tolerance appeared progressively and was found to be statistically significant after 2 weeks of treatment. The parameters used by Beauge et al. [168] to measure the development of tolerance included the hypothermic response and motor performance on a tilting plane following a challenge dose of ethanol. Simultaneously with the development of tolerance, they observed a slight but progressively increasing augmentation of the basal synaptosomal Na^+/K^+ ATPase activity. In nonwithdrawn animals, they found that the norepinephrine-ethanol interaction was markedly reduced in comparison with controls. This confirms previous work suggesting that norepinephrine sensitizes Na^+/K^+ ATPase [169,170] to ethanol. These results also support the view that the changes in the ethanol-treated group are associated with the development of tolerance rather than being the consequences of withdrawal. Furthermore, their data show that the time course in the reduction of the norepinephrine-ethanol interaction correlated positively with the time course of the development of functional tolerance. Their results support the hypothesis that ethanol-induced alterations of Na^+/K^+ ATPase activity may be related to the development of tolerance to ethanol, although the underlying mechanisms require further elucidation.

As suggested by Beauge et al. [171], the simultaneity of development of various physical, biochemical, and functional alterations during ethanol intoxication support the concept that these parameters represent different aspects of a single phenomenon, i.e. tolerance to ethanol. Their results indicate that the fluidizing and Na^+/K^+ ATPase activity effects of ethanol added *in vitro* are consistent and meaningful for tolerance analyses. Membranes from ethanol-treated rats were found to be less responsive than those from control animals.

11.4.3 Alterations in Ca^{2+}/Mg^{2+} ATPase. Garrett and Ross [172] observed that acute administration of ethanol in mice inhibited Ca^{2+}/Mg^{2+} ATPase and ATP-dependent Ca^{2+} uptake into endoplasmic reticulum-like organelles in synaptosomal membranes. The changes observed correlated with loss and recovery of the righting reflex.

12 CLINICAL USES OF ETHANOL THAT MAY AFFECT SYNAPTOGENESIS

The potential dangers of ethanol exposure during this ontogenetic period seem not to be fully appreciated, as evidenced by the clinical uses of ethanol, particularly during the past two decades. The benefits versus the potential dangers should be carefully evaluated.

12.1 Obstetrical Use of Ethanol

Recently Landesman-Dwyer [173] reviewed the obstetrical use of ethanol, and found that it had been used to some extent for control of pain associated with labor [174,175]. However, if administered too early ethanol was found to cause a decrease in the frequency and strength of uterine contractions or to cause total cessation of labor [174,175].

In more recent years ethanol was introduced for use in the inhibition of premature labor [176–181], and it continues to be included among the pharmacological inhibitors of premature labor or oxytocin-induced term labor [182–193]. Although selective β_2-agonists are useful for inhibition of premature labor [194], the intravenous use of ethanol for this purpose has not been completely abandoned.

Sisenwein et al. [195] reported that a subgroup of children born during or within 15 h of termination of ethanol infusion showed significant pathology upon developmental testing and personality inventory at ages 4–7 years. Landesman-Dwyer [173] pointed out that behavioral assessment of children born of mothers who had received ethanol intravenously was extremely limited.

12.2 Pediatric Use of Ethanol

Another clinical use of ethanol was in hyperalimentation in small-for-dates infants. The dangers of infantile intoxication during hyperalimentation in small-for-dates infants was pointed out by Peden et al. [196]. They observed that infants receiving this treatment were lethargic and they found BECs as high as 163–183 mg/dl in several infants. Cook et al. [179] also stressed the possible dangers associated with the addition of ethanol to hyperalimentation solutions for use in treatment of small-for-dates infants.

These recent clinical uses of ethanol to control pain during term labor, to inhibit premature labor, or to provide hyperalimentation feedings in small-for-dates infants indicates a lack of awareness of the potential dangers of ethanol exposure during the brain growth spurt. This underlines the importance of research concerning the effects of ethanol on the developing brain, particularly during the brain growth spurt.

The notion that ethanol in "moderate" amounts is not harmful to the mother or the conceptus, particularly during the late stages of pregnancy, may have been confirmed to some extent by these clinical uses of ethanol, despite widely publicized information relative to the occurrence of the FAS in infants born of alcoholic women. It is of crucial importance that information relative to the potential dangers of ethanol exposure during the brain growth spurt be disseminated not only to parents and future parents but also to health care professionals.

13 LEVEL OF AWARENESS OF ALCOHOL-RELATED PROBLEMS

Dedication of the October 12, 1984, issue of the Journal of the American Medical Association (JAMA) to alcoholism and related problems is a landmark contribution of the American Medical Association (AMA). As pointed out by Niven [197], nearly 30 years ago the AMA House of Delegates, in 1956, issued a statement recognizing that alcoholism is an illness that comes within the scope of medical practice. The AMA's Manual on Alcoholism was first published in 1968 and has been revised several times. In 1982, the AMA's Panel on Alcoholism within the AMA Council on Scientific Affairs adopted a report and recommendation relative to the FAS [198].

According to Niven [197] a poll conducted recently by the AMA indicates that physicians almost unanimously recognize alcoholism as a major national and international problem. However, only 27% of the respondents answered that they felt competent to treat alcoholic patients. Undoubtedly this special issue of JAMA, widely subscribed to by physicians, will heighten awareness of this group concerning the seriousness of alcohol-related problems. The most important paper included in the issue that is relevant to the effects of ethanol during the brain growth spurt is that of Mills and colleagues [135], which indicates that birth weight in infants decreased with increasing maternal alcohol intake.

14 QUESTIONABLE SAFETY OF DRINKING DURING PREGNANCY

In spite of numerous studies, there has been no consensus as to whether moderate social drinking is harmful to an unborn infant. Mills and colleagues [135] reported on a prospective study in which they had collected data from 31,604 pregnancies during the years 1974—1977. They found that the percentage of newborns below the tenth percentile of weight for gestational age increased sharply with increasing maternal alcohol intake. Furthermore, they found that consuming one or two drinks daily was associated with a substantially increased risk of producing a growth-retarded infant. These authors pointed out that a safe level of alcohol intake that will not cause malformations has not been established. They advised that pregnant women limit themselves to an "occasional" drink and stated that they do not recommend that pregnant women be told that any drinking, unless it is less than one drink per day, is safe. The data collected in their study did not permit assessment of binge drinking. Further, data collection was limited to the first trimester of pregnancy. Does this indicate an unawareness on the part of researchers that maternal ethanol intake during the second and third trimesters may pose a threat to the developing brain?

15 CONCLUSIONS

The most devastating effects of ethanol on fetal outcome are undoubtedly due to maternal alcoholism *per se.* The neuropathology associated with the full-blown FAS probably arises during the first trimester of human pregnancy. However, attention deficit disorder, hyperactivity, and related difficulties in learning may be among the more subtle though serious effects of synaptic neuropathology that are likely to be induced by a relatively low-intensity ethanol exposure during synaptogenesis.

Ethanol-induced alteration in synaptic membrane fluidity, or in the molecular structure of the pre- and postsynaptic membranes during synaptogenesis, is likely to affect processes involved in recognition and adhesion mechanisms that are essential to the establishment of synaptic connections. These changes may not be visible at the light or electron microscope levels but may be detectable biochemically. More important, changes at this level may be reflected in developmental cognitive and behavioral disorders.

16 ACKNOWLEDGMENTS

The author is indebted to Tom W. Kruckeberg, Mary F. Kanak, Catherine J. Keys, Virginia M. Dress, and Amy L. Shoemaker for helpful assistance in the preparation of this manuscript.

17 REFERENCES

1. Jones KL, Smith DW: Recognition of the fetal alcohol syndrome in early infancy. Lancet 2:999–1001, 1973.
2. Jones KL, Smith DW, Ulleland CN, Striessguth AP: Pattern of malformation in offspring of chronic alcoholic mothers. Lancet 1:1267–1271, 1973.
3. Jones KL, Smith DW, Streissguth AP, Myrianthopoulos NC: Outcome in offspring of chronic alcoholic women. Lancet 1:2076–2078, 1974.

4. Warren KR: "Critical Review of the Fetal Alcohol Syndrome." National Institute of Alcohol Abuse and Alcoholism. Available through the National Clearinghouse for Alcohol Information, PO Box 2345, Rockville, Maryland, 20852, 1977.
5. Clarren SK, Alvord EC, Sumi SM, Streissguth AP, Smith DW: Brain malformations related to prenatal exposure to ethanol. J Pediatr 92:64–67, 1978.
6. Alpert JJ, Day N, Dooling E, Hingson R, Oppenheimer, E, Rosett HL, Weiner L, Zukerman B: Maternal alcohol consumption and newborn assessment: Methodology of the Boston City Hospital prospective study. Neurobehav Toxicol Teratol 3:187–194, 1981.
7. Landesman-Dwyer S, Ragozin AS: Behavioral correlates of prenatal alcohol exposure: A four-year follow-up study. Neurobehav Toxicol Teratol 3:187–194, 1981.
8. Colangelo W, Jones DG: The fetal alcohol syndrome: A review and assessment of the syndrome and its neurological sequelae. Prog Neurobiol 19:271–314, 1982.
9. Ouellette EM, Rosett HL, Rosman NP, Winer L: Adverse effects on offspring of maternal alcohol abuse during pregnancy. N Engl J Med 297:528, 1977.
10. Sokol RJ, Miller SI, Reed G: Alcohol abuse during pregnancy: An epidemiologic study. Alcoholism. Clin Exp Res 4:135–145, 1980.
11. Hanson JW, Streissguth AP, Smith DW: The effects of moderate alcohol consumption during pregnancy on fetal growth and morphogenesis. J Pediatr 92:457, 1978.
12. Shaywitz BA, Griffieth GG, Warshaw JB: Hyperactivity and cognitive deficits in developing rat pups born to alcoholic mothers: An experimental model of the expanded fetal alcohol syndrome (EFAS). Neurobehav Toxicol 1:113–122, 1979.
13. Clarren SK, Smith DW: The fetal alcohol syndrome. N Engl J Med 298:1063–1067, 1978.
14. Timiras PS, Vernadakis A, Sherwood NM: Development and plasticity of the nervous system. In Assali NS (ed): "Biology of Gestation." New York: Academic, 1968, pp 261–319.
15. Vernadakis A, Woodbury DM: The developing animal as a model. Epilepsia 10:163–178, 1969.
16. Altman J: Postnatal development of the cerebellar cortex in the rat: I. The external germinal layer and the transitional molecular layer. J Comp Neurol 145:353–398, 1972.
17. Altman J: Postnatal development of the cerebellar cortex in the rat: II. Phases in the maturation of purkinje cells and of the molecular layer. J Comp Neurol 145:399–464, 1972.
18. Altman J: Postnatal development of the cerebellar cortex in the rat: III. Maturation of the components of the granular layer. J Comp Neurol 145:465–514, 1972.
19. Altman J: Autoradiographic and histological studies of postnatal neurogenesis: III. Dating the time of production and onset of differentiation of cerebellar microneurons in rats. J Comp Neurol 136:269–294, 1969.
20. Ito M: Purkinje cells: Morphology and development. "The Cerebellum and Neural Control." New York: Raven, 1984, pp 21–39.
21. Del Cerro MP, Snider RS: Studies on the developing cerebellum: Ultrastructure of the growth cones. J Comp Neurol 133:341–362, 1968.
22. Gottlieb A, Keydar I, Epstein HT: Rodent brain growth stages: An analytical review. Biol Neonate 32:166–176, 1977.
23. Moore KL: "The Developing Human: Clinically Oriented Embryology." 2nd ed. Philadelphia: W.A. Saunders, 1977, pp 33–95; 319–358.

24. Lemire RJ, Loeser JD, Leech RW, Alvord EC Jr: "Normal and Abnormal Development of the Human Nervous System." Hagerstown, MD: Harper and Row, 1975.
25. Dobbing J: The later growth of the brain and its vulnerability. Pediatrics 53:2–6, 1974.
26. Dobbing J: Undernutrition and the developing brain. In Paoletti R, Davison AN (eds): "Chemistry and Brain Development. Advances in Experimental Medicine and Biology, 13." New York: Plenum, 1971, pp 399–412.
27. Dobbing J, Smart JL: Early undernutrition, brain development and behavior. In Barnett SA (ed): "Ethology and Development. Clinics in Developmental Medicine, 47." Philadelphia: Lippincott, 1973, pp 16–36.
28. Dobbing J, Sands J: Comparative aspects of the brain growth spurt. Early Hum Dev 3:79–83, 1979.
29. Cotman CW, Nieto-Sampedro: Cell biology of synaptic plasticity. Science 225:1287–1294, 1984.
30. Black IB, Adler JE, Dreyfus CF, Jonakait GM, Katz DM, KaGamma EF, Markey KM: Neurotransmitter plasticity at the molecular level. Science 225:1266–1270, 1984.
31. Burry RW, Kniss DA, Scribner LR: Mechanisms of synapse formation and maturation. In Jones DG (ed): "Current Topics in Research on Synapses, 1." New York: Alan R. Liss, 1984, pp 1–51.
32. Fox HE, Steinbrecher M, Pressel D, Inglis J, Medvid L, Angel E: Maternal ethanol ingestion and the occurrence of human fetal breathing movements. Am J Obstet Gynecol 132:354–358, 1978.
33. Le AV, Doyle D: General theory of membrane structure and function. In Venter JCR, Harrison LC (eds): "Membranes, Detergents, and Receptor Solubilization." New York: Alan R. Liss, 1984, pp 1–25.
34. Robertson JD: Review of membrane structure with perspectives on certain transmembrane channels. In Waxman SG, Ritchie JM (eds): "Demyelinating Disease: Basic and Clinical Electrophysiology." New York: Raven, 1981, pp 419–477.
35. Pfenninger KH: Organization of neuronal membranes. Annu Rev Neurosci 1:445–471, 1978.
36. Morgan IG, Gombos G: Biochemical studies of synaptic macromolecules. In Barondes SH (ed): "Neuronal Recognition." New York: Plenum, 1976, pp 179–202.
37. Pfenninger KH, Maylie-Pfenninger MF: Properties and dynamics of plasmalemmal glycoconjugates in growing neurites. In Cuenod M, Kreutzberg GW, Gloom FE (eds): "Development and Chemical Specificity of Neurons. Progress in Brain Research, 51." Amsterdam: Elsevier/North-Holland, 1979, pp 83–94.
38. Edelman GM: Surface modulation in cell recognition and cell growth. Some new hypotheses on phenotypic alteration and transmembranous control of cell surface receptors. Science 192:218–226, 1976.
39. Pfenninger KH, Rees RP: From the growth cone to the synapse. Properties of membranes involved in synapse formation. In Barondes SH (ed): "Neuronal Recognition." New York: Plenum, 1976, pp 131–178.
40. Barondes SH: Brain glycomacromolecules and interneuronal recognition. In Schmitt FO (ed): "The Neurosciences." New York: Rockefeller University Press, 1970, pp 747–760.
41. Small RK, Pfenninger KH: Components of the plasma membrane of growing axons. I. Size and distribution of intramembrane particles. J Cell Biol 98:1422–1433, 1984.

42. Small RK, Blank M, Ghez R, Pfenninger KH: Components of the plasma membrane of growing axons. II. Diffusion of membrane protein complexes. J Cell Biol 98:1434–1443, 1984.
43. Pfenninger KH, Maylie-Pfenninger MF: Lectin labeling of sprouting neurons. I. Regional distribution of surface glycoconjugates. J Cell Biol 89:536–546, 1981.
44. Pfenninger KH, Johnson MP: Membrane biogenesis in the sprouting neuron. I. Selective transfer of newly synthesized phospholipid into the growing neurite. J Cell Biol 97:1038–1042, 1983.
45. Pfenninger KH, Maylie-Pfenninger MF: Lectin labeling of sprouting neurons. II. Relative movement and appearance of glycoconjugates during plasmalemmal expansion. J Cell Biol 89:547–559, 1981.
46. Pfenninger KH, Ellis L, Johnson MP, Friedman LB, Somlo S: Nerve growth cones isolated from fetal rat brain: Subcellular fractionation and characterization. Cell 35:573–584, 1983.
47. Strichartz GR, Small RK, Pfenninger KH: Components of the plasma membrane of growing axons. III. Saxitoxin binding to sodium channels. J Cell Biol 98:1444–1452, 1984.
48. Goodman CS, Bastiani MJ, Doe CQ, du Lac S, Helfand SL, Kuwada JY, Thomas JB: Cell recognition during neuronal development. Science 225:1271–1279, 1984.
49. Babitch JA: Synaptic plasma membrane tubulin may be an integral constituent. J Neurochem 37:1394–1400, 1981.
50. Hitzemann RJ, Harris RA: Developmental changes in synaptic membrane fluidity: A comparison of 1,6-diphenyl-1,3,5,-hexatriene (DPH) and 1-4[4-(trimethylamino)-phenyl]-6-phenyl-1,3,5,-hexatriene (TMA-DPH). Dev Brain Res 14:113–120, 1984.
51. Caley DW, Maxwell DS: Ultrastructure of the developing cerebral cortex in the rat. In Sterman MB, McGinty DS, Adinolfi AM (eds): "Brain Development and Behavior." New York: Academic, 1971, pp 91–107.
52. Johnson DA, Lee NM, Cooke R, Loh HH: Ethanol-induced fluidization of brain lipid bilayers: Required presence of cholesterol in membranes for the expression of tolerance. Mol Pharmacol 15:739–746, 1979.
53. Thiery J-P, Duband J-L, Rutishauser U, Edelman GM: Cell adhesion molecules in early chick embryogenesis. Proc Natl Acad Sci USA 79:6737–6741, 1982.
54. Rothbard JB, Brackenbury R, Cunningham BA, Edelman GM: Differences in the carbohydrate structures of neural cell-adhesion molecules from adult and embryonic chicken brains. J Biol Chem 257:11064–11069, 1982.
55. Stibler H, Burns EM, Kruckeberg TW, Gaetano PK, Cerven E, Borg S, Tabakoff B: Effect of ethanol on synaptosomal sialic acid metabolism in the developing rat brain. J Neurol Sci 59:21–35, 1983.
56. Edelman GM: Cell adhesion molecules. Science 219:450–457, 1983.
57. Caviness VS, Rakic P: Mechanisms of cortical development: A view from mutations in mice. Annu Rev Neurosci 1:297–326, 1978.
58. Roth S, McGuire EJ, Roseman S: Evidence for cell-surface glycosyltransferases: Their potential role in cell surface recognition. J Cell Biol 51:536–547, 1971.
59. Brunngraber EG: Brief proposals. The possible role of glycoproteins in neural function. Perspect Biol Med 12:467–470, 1969.
60. Roseman S: Synthesis of complex carbohydrates by multi-glucosyltransferase systems and their potential function in intercellular adhesion. Chem Phys Lipids 5:270–297, 1970.

61. Morgan DG, Routtenberg A: Incorporation of intrastriatally injected (3H)fructose into electrophoretically separated synaptosomal glycoproteins. I. Turnover and molecular weight estimations. Brain Res 179:329–341, 1979.
62. Brunngraber EG: Glycoproteins in neural tissue. In Lajtha A (ed): "Protein Metabolism of the Nervous System." New York: Plenum, 1970, pp 383–407.
63. Mena EE, Foster AC, Fagg GE, Cotman, CW: Identification of synapse specific components: Synaptic glycoproteins, proteins, and transmitter binding sites. J Neurochem 37:1557–1566, 1981.
64. Mena EE, Cotman CW: Synaptic cleft glycoproteins contain homologous amino acid sequences. Science 216:422–424, 1982.
65. Sperry RW: Chemoaffinity in the orderly growth of nerve fiber patterns and connections. Proc Natl Acad Sci USA 50:703–710, 1963.
66. Jacobson M: Development, specification, and diversification of neural connections. In Schmitt FO (ed): "The Neurosciences: Second Study Program." New York: Rockefeller University Press, 1970, pp 116–129.
67. Fu SC, Cruz TF, Gurd JW: Development of synaptic glycoproteins: Effect of postnatal age on the synthesis and concentration of synaptic membrane and synaptic junctional fucosyl and sialyl glycoproteins. J Neurochem 36:1338–1351, 1981.
68. Cruz TF, Gurd JW: Effect of development on activity, specificity and endogenous substrates of synaptic membrane sialidase. Biochim Biophys Acta 675:201–208, 1981.
69. Cruz TF, Gurd JW: Developmental changes in the biosynthesis of sialoglycoprotein substrates for intrinsic synaptic sialidase. J Neurochem 40:1487–1489, 1983.
70. Mintz G, Gottlieb DI, Reitman ML, Derby M, Glaser L: Development changes in glycoproteins of the chick nervous system. Brain Res 206:51–70, 1981.
71. Federico A, DiBenedetta C: Glycoprotein changes during the development of human brain. J Neurochem 31:797–800, 1978.
72. Van Den Eijnden DH, Van Dijk W, Roukema PA: Sialoglycoprotein synthesis in developing rat brain. Neurobiology 5:221–227, 1975.
73. Suzuki K: Pattern of mammalian brain gangliosides. III. Regional and development differences. J Neurochem 12:969–979, 1965.
74. Ledeen R, Yu RK: Gangliosides as constituents of nervous system membranes. In Bogoch S (ed): "Biological Diagnosis of Brain Disorders." New York: Spectrum, 1973, pp 247–257.
75. Svennerholm L: Gangliosides and synaptic transmission. Adv Exp Med Biol 125:533–544, 1980.
76. Hess HH, Bass NH, Thalheimer C, Devarakonda R: Gangliosides and the architecture of human frontal cortex and rat somatosensory isocortex. J Neurochem 26:1115–1121, 1976.
77. Bass NH: Ganglioside sialic acid as a quantitative neurochemical index of the integrity of synaptic function in cognitive disorders of development and aging. In Rapport MM, Gorio A (eds): "Gangliosides in Neurological and Neuromuscular Function and Repair." New York: Raven, 1981, pp 29–43.
78. Hess HH, Pope A: Quantitative neurochemical histology. In Lajtha A (ed): "Handbook of Neurochemistry." New York: Plenum, 1971, Vol 7, pp 289–327.
79. Lund RD: "Development and Plasticity of the Brain." New York: Oxford University Press, 1978.
80. Santini M (ed): "Golgi Centennial Symposium: Perspectives in Neurobiology." New York: Raven, 1975.

81. Dreyfus H, Harth S, Yusufi ANK, Urban PR, Mandel P: Sialyltransferase activities in two neuronal models: Retina and cultures of isolated neurons. Adv Exp Med Biol 125:227–238, 1980.
82. Ng SS, Dain JA: Sialyltransferases in rat brain: Reaction kinetics, product analyses, and multiplicities of enzyme species. J Neurochem 29:1075–1083, 1977.
83. Duffard RO, Capputo R: A natural inhibitor of sialyltransferase and its possible influence on this enzyme activity during brain development. Biochemistry 11:1396–1400, 1972.
84. Van Den Eijnden DH, Van Dijk W: Properties and regional distribution of cerebral CMP-N-acetylneuraminic acid: Glycoprotein sialyltransferase. Biochim Biophys Acta 362:136–149, 1974.
85. Preti A, Fiorilli A, Lombardo A, Caimi L, Tettamanti G: Occurrence of sialyltransferase activity in the synaptosomal membranes prepared from calf brain cortex. J Neurochem 33:281–296, 1980.
86. Baumann H, Doyle D: Determination of carbohydrate structures in glycoproteins and glycolipids. In Venter JC, Harrison LC (eds): "Molecular and Chemical Characterization of Membrane Receptors." New York: Alan R. Liss, 1984, pp 125–160.
87. Samson HH, Diaz J: Effects of neonatal ethanol exposure on brain development in rodents. In Abel EL (ed): "Fetal Alcohol Syndrome. Vol 3. Animal Studies." Boca Raton, FL: CRC Press, 1981, pp 131–150.
88. West JR, Hodges-Savola CA: Permanent hippocampal mossy fiber hyperdevelopment following prenatal ethanol exposure. Neurobehav Toxicol Teratol 5:139–150, 1983.
89. Pierce DR, Hamre KM, West JR: Ethanol exposure alters hippocampal development during the brain growth spurt in rats. Abstr Soc Neurosci 10:248, 1984.
90. Adlard BPF, Dobbing J, Smart JL: An alternative animal model for the full-term small-for-dates human baby. Biol Neonate 23:95–108, 1973.
91. Dobbing J: The later development of the brain and its vulnerability. In Davis JA, Dobbing J (eds): "Scientific Foundations of Paediatrics." Philadelphia: WB Saunders, 1974, pp 565–577.
92. Rawat AK: Ribosomal protein synthesis in the fetal and neonatal brain as influenced by ethanol consumption. Res Commun Chem Pathol Pharmacol 12:723–732, 1975.
93. Abel EL: Emotionality in offspring of rats fed alcohol while nursing. J Stud Alcohol 36:654–658, 1975.
94. Martin JC, Martin DC, Sigman G, Radow B: Offspring survival, development and operant performance following ethanol consumption. Dev Psychobiol 10:435–446, 1977.
95. Yanai J, Ginsburg BE: Long-term reduction of male agnostic behavior in mice following early exposure to ethanol. Psychopharmacology 52:31–34, 1977.
96. Bond NW: Postnatal alcohol exposure in the rat: Its effects on avoidance conditioning, Hebb-Williams maze performance, maternal behavior, and pup development. Physiol Psychol 8:437–443, 1980.
97. Wiener SG, Shoemaker WJ, Koda LY, Bloom FE: Interaction of ethanol and nutrition during gestation: Influence on maternal and offspring development in the rat. J Pharmacol Exp Ther 216:572–579, 1981.
98. Abel EL: Procedural considerations in evaluating prenatal effects of alcohol in animals. Neurobehav Toxicol 2:167–174, 1980.
99. Phillips SC, Cragg BG: A change in susceptibility of rat cerebellar Purkinje cells to damage by alcohol during fetal, neonatal and adult life. Neuropathol Appl Neurobiol 8:441–454, 1982.

100. Bauer-Moffett C, Altman J: The effect of ethanol chronically administered to preweanling rats on cerebellar development: A morphological study. Brain Res 119:249–268, 1977.
101. Diaz J, Samson HH: Impaired brain growth in neonatal rats exposed to ethanol. Science 208:751–753, 1980.
102. Diaz J, Moore E, Petracca F, Schacher J, Stamper C: Artificial rearing of preweanling rats: The effectiveness of direct intragastric feeding. Physiol Behav 27:1103–1105, 1981.
103. Samson HH, Grant KA, Coggan S, Sachs VM: Ethanol induced microcephaly in the neonatal rat: Occurrence without withdrawal. Neurobehav Toxicol 4:115–116, 1982.
104. West JR, Dewey SL, Pierce DR, Black AC Jr: Prenatal and early postnatal exposure to ethanol permanently alters the rat hippocampus. In Porter R, O'Connor M, Whelan J (eds); "Mechanisms of Alcohol Damage in Utero." Ciba Foundation Symposium, 105. London: Pittman, 1984, pp 8–25.
105. Grant KA, Choi EY, Samson HH: Neonatal ethanol exposure: Effects on adult behavior and brain growth parameters. Pharmacol Biochem Behav 18(Suppl 1):331–336, 1983.
106. Hall WG: Weaning and growth of artificially reared rats. Science 190:1313–1315, 1975.
107. Messer M, Thoman EB, Galofre A, Dallman T, Dallman P: Artificial feeding of infant rats by continuous gastric infusion. J Nutr 98:404–410, 1969.
108. Diamond MG, Rosenzweig MR, Bennett EL, Lindner B, Lyon L: Effects of environmental enrichment and impoverishment on rat cerebral cortex. J Neurobiol 3:47–64, 1972.
109. Diamaond MC, Ingham CA, Johnson RE, Bennett EL, Rosenzweig MR: Effects of environment on morphology of rat cerebral cortex and hippocampus. J Neurobiol 7:75–85, 1976.
110. Greenough WT, Volkman FR, Juraska JM: Effects of rearing complexity on dendritic branching in frontolateral and temporal cortex of the rat. Exp Neurol 41:371–378, 1973.
111. Greenough WT, West RW, DeVoogd TJ: Synaptic plate perforations: Changes with age and experience in the rat. Science 202:1096–1098, 1978.
112. Wesa JM, Chang F-LF, Greenough WT, West RW: Synaptic contact curvature: Effects of differential rearing on rat occipital cortex. Dev Brain Res 4:253–257, 1982.
113. Burns EM, Kruckeberg TW, Kanak MF, Stibler H: Postnatal ethanol exposure: Permanent central nervous system effects. Fed Proc 43:494, 1984.
114. Bauer-Moffett C, Altman J: Ethanol-induced reductions in cerebellar growth of infant rats. Exp Neurol 48:378–382, 1975.
115. Barnes DE, Walker DW: Prenatal ethanol exposure permanently reduces the number of pyramidal neurons in rat hippocampus. Dev Brain Res 1:333–340, 1981.
116. Borges S, Lewis PD: A study of alcohol effects on the brain during gestation and lactation. Teratology 25:283–289, 1982.
117. Burns EM, Kruckeberg TW, Stibler H, Cerven E, Borg S: Ethanol exposure during brain growth spurt in rats. Teratology 29:251–258, 1984.
118. Jones DG, Colangelo W: An ultrastructural investigation into the influence of ethanol on synaptic maturation in rat neocortex. I. Qualitative assessment. Dev Neurosci 7:94–106, 1985.

119. Jones DG, Colangelo W: An ultrastructural investigation into the influence of ethanol on synaptic maturation in rat neocortex. II. Quantitative analysis. Dev Neurosci 7:107–119, 1985.
120. Yanai J, Ginsburg BE: Audiogenic seizures in mice whose parents drank alcohol. J Stud Alcohol 37:1564–1571, 1976.
121. Sonderegger T, Colburn D, Calmers H, Corbitt S, Zimmerman E: Methodological note: Intragastric intubation of ethanol to rat pups. Neurobehav Toxicol Teratol 4:477–481, 1982.
122. Klemm WR: Ethanol tolerance: Evidence of "protective" effects on brains of adult rats. J Neurosci Res 3:353–358, 1978.
123. Klemm WR, Engen RL: Biochemical markers of ethanol effects on brain. J Neurosci Res 3:341–351, 1978.
124. Klemm WR, Engen RL: Acutely administered ethanol decreases whole-brain sialic acid and cerebellar 2-deoxyribose. J Neurosci Res 4:371–382, 1979.
125. Klemm WR, Engen RL: Effects of ethanol on brain sialic acid and 2-deoxyribose in young rats. J Stud Alcohol 40:554–561,, 1979.
126. Lehninger AL: "Biochemistry." New York: Worth, 1968, pp 506–507.
127. Rahmann H, Rosner H, Breer H: A functional model of the sialoglycomacromolecules in synaptic transmission and memory formation. J Theor Biol 57:231, 1976.
128. Bosman HB: Synthesis of glycoproteins in brain: Identification, purification and properties of glycosyltransferases from purified synaptosomes of guinea pig cerebral cortex. J Neurochem 19:763–778, 1972.
129. Yamakawa T, Nagai Y: Glycolipids at the cell surface and their biological function. Trends Biochem Sci 3:128–131, 1978.
130. Tauc L, Hinzen D: Neuraminidase: Its effect on synaptic transmission. Brain Res 80:340–344, 1974.
131. Stibler H, Burns EM, Kruckeberg TW, Cerven E, Borg S: Changes of synaptosomal surface carbohydrates after ethanol exposure during synaptogenesis. In Parvez H, Burns EM, Burov Y, Parvez S (eds): "Alcohol, Nutrition, and the Nervous System." Utrecht, Holland: VNU International Science Press (in press).
132. Kruckeberg TW, Gaetano PK, Burns EM, Stibler H, Cerven E, Borg S: Ethanol in preweanling rats with dams: Body temperature unaffected. Neurobehav Toxicol Teratol 6:307–312, 1984.
133. Littleton J: Development of membrane tolerance to ethanol may limit intoxication and influence dependence liability. In Sandler M (ed): "Psychcopharmacology of Alcohol." New York: Raven, 1980, pp 121–127.
134. Majchrowicz E, Hunt WA: Temporal relationship of the induction of tolerance and physical dependence after continuous intoxication with maximum tolerable doses of ethanol in rats. Psychopharmacology 50:107–112, 1976.
135. Mills JL, Graubard BI, Harley EE, Rhoads GG, Berendes HW: Maternal alcohol consumption and birth weight: How much drinking during pregnancy is safe? J Am Med Assoc 252:1875–1879, 1984.
136. Majchrowicz E: Reversal in central nervous system function during ethanol withdrawal in humans and experimental animals. Fed Proc 40:2065-2072, 1981.
137. Majchrowicz E, Hunt WA: Neurobiological correlates of intoxication and physical dependence upon ethanol. Introductory remarks. Fed Proc 40:2048–2050, 1981.
138. Blakley PM, Scott WJ Jr: Determination of the proximate teratogen of the mouse fetal alcohol syndrome. Toxicol Appl Pharmacol 72:355–363, 1984.

139. Le Bourhis B, Aufrere G: Alcohol exposure pattern and physical dependence. Pharmacol Biochem Behav 18(Suppl 1):511–514, 1983.
140. Chin JH, Goldstein DB: Effects of low concentrations of ethanol on the fluidity of spin-labelled erythrocyte and brain membranes. Mol Pharmacol 13:435–441, 1977.
141. Chin JH, Goldstein DB: Drug tolerance in biomembranes: A spin label study of the effects of ethanol. Science 196:684–685, 1977.
142. Goldstein DB, Chin JH: Interaction of ethanol with biological membranes. Fed Proc 40:2073–2076, 1981.
143. Goldstein DB: The effects of drugs on membrane fluidity. Annu Rev Pharmacol Toxicol 24:43–64, 1984.
144. Goldstein DB, Hungund BL, Lyon RC: Increased surface glycoconjugates of synaptic membranes in mice during chronic ethanol treatment. Br J Pharmacol 78:8–10, 1983.
145. Johnson DA, Friedman HJ, Cooke R, Lee NM: Adaptation of brain lipid bilayers to ethanol-induced fluidization. Biochem Pharmacol 29:1673–1676, 1980.
146. Logan BJ, Laverty R, Peake BM: ESR measurements on the effects of ethanol on the lipid and protein conformation in biological membranes. Pharmacol Biochem Behav 18(Suppl 1):31–35, 1983.
147. Crews FT, Majchrowicz E, Meeks R: Changes in cortical synaptosomal plasma membrane fluidity and composition in ethanol-dependent rats. Psychopharmacology 81:208–213, 1983.
148. Smith TL, Gerhart MJ: Alteration in brain lipid composition of mice made physically dependent to ethanol. Life Sci 31:1419–1425, 1982.
149. Lee NM, Friedman HJ, Loh HH: Effect of acute and chronic ethanol treatment on rat brain phospholipid turnover. Biochem Pharmacol 29:2815–2818, 1980.
150. Harris RA, Groh GI, Baxter DM, Hitzemann RJ: Gangliosides enhance the membrance actions of ethanol and pentobarbitol. Mol Pharmacol 25:410–417, 1984.
151. Sun GY, Sun AY: Chronic ethanol administration induced an increase in phosphatidylserine in guinea pig synaptic plasma membranes. Biochem Biophys Res Commun 113:262–268, 1983.
152. Rubin E, Rottenberg H: Ethanol and biological membranes: Injury and adaptation. Pharmacol Biochem Behav 18(Suppl 1):7–13, 1983.
153. Harris RA, Schroeder F: Ethanol and the physical properties of brain membranes. Mol Pharmacol 20:128–137, 1981.
154. Harris RA, Hood WF: Inhibition of synaptosomal calcium uptake by ethanol. J Pharmacol Exp Ther 213:562–568, 1980.
155. Harris RA, Fenner D: Ethanol and synaptosomal calcium binding. Biochem Pharmacol 31:1790–1792, 1982.
156. Stokes JA, Harris RA: Alcohol and synaptosomal calcium transport. Mol Pharmacol 22:99–104, 1982.
157. Burke JP, Tumbleson ME, Seaman RN, Sun AY: Alcohol-membrane interaction: Calcium uptake in mitochondria. Res Commun Chem Pathol Pharmacol 18:569–572, 1977.
158. Michaelis ML, Michaelis EK, Tehan T: Alcohol effects on synaptic membrane calcium ion fluxes. Pharmacol Biochem Behav 18(Suppl 1):19–23, 1983.
159. Guerri C, Grisolia S: Chronic ethanol treatment affects synaptosomal membrane-bound enzymes. Pharmacol Biochem Behav 18(Suppl 1):45–50, 1983.
160. Rabin RA, Molinoff PB: Multiple sites of action of ethanol on adenylate cyclase. J Pharmacol Exp Ther 227:551–556, 1983.

161. Luthin GR, Tabakoff B: Activation of adenylate cyclase by alcohols requires the nucleotide-binding protein. J Pharmacol Exp Ther 228:579–587, 1984.
162. Israel Y, Kalant H, LeBlanc E, Berstein JC, Salazar I: Changes in cation transport and Na^+/K^+ activated adenosine triphosphatase produced by chronic administration of ethanol. J Pharmacol Exp Ther 174:330–336, 1970.
163. Seeman P: The membrane actions of anesthetics and tranquilizers. Pharmacol Rev 24:583–645, 1972.
164. Levental M, Tabakoff B: Sodium-potassium-activated adenosine triphosphatase activity as a measure of neuronal membrane characteristics in ethanol-tolerant mice. J Pharmacol Exp Ther 212:315–319, 1980.
165. Roach MK: Changes in the activity of (Na^+ and K^+)ATPase during acute and chronic administration of ethanol. In Majchrowicz E, Noble EP (eds): "Biochemistry and Pharmacology of Ethanol." New York: Plenum, Vol 2, 1979.
166. Beauge F, Fleuret-Balter C, Barin F, Nordmann J, Nordmann R: Brain membrane disordering related to acute ethanol administration in naive and short-term ethanol-intoxicated rats. Drug Alcohol Depend 10:143–151, 1982.
167. Fleuret-Balter C, Beauge F, Barin F, Nordmann J, Nordmann R: Brain membrane disordering by administration of a single ethanol dose. Pharmacol Biochem Behav 18:25–29, 1983.
168. Beauge F, Stibler H, Kalant H: Brain synaptosomal (Na^+/K^+)ATPase activity as an index of tolerance to ethanol. Pharmacol Biochem Behav 18:519–524, 1983
169. Rangaraj N, Kalant H: Effects of ethanol withdrawal, stress and amphetamine on rat brain (Na^+ and K^+)-ATPase. Biochem Pharmacol 27:1139–1144, 1978.
170. Rangaraj N, Kalant H: Acute and chronic catecholamine-ethanol interaction on rat brain (Na^+ and K^+)-ATPase. Pharmacol Biochem Behav 13(Suppl 1):183–189, 1980.
171. Beauge F, Fleuret-Balter C, Nordmann J, Nordmann R: Brain membrane sensitivity to ethanol during development of functional tolerance to ethanol in rats. Alcoholism: Clin Exp Res 8:167–171, 1984.
172. Garrett KM, Ross DH: Effects of in vivo ethanol administration on Ca^{2+}/Mg^{2+} ATPase and ATP-dependent Ca^{2+} uptake activity in synaptosomes. Neurochem Res 8:1013–1028, 1983.
173. Landesman-Dwyer S: The relationship of children's behavior to maternal alcohol consumption. In Abel AL (ed): "Fetal Alcohol Syndrome." Boca Raton, FL: CRC Press, 1981, Vol 2, pp 127–148.
174. Belinkoff S, Hall OW Jr: Intravenous alcohol during labor. Am J Obstet Gynecol 59:429, 1950.
175. Chapman ER, Williams PT: Intravenous alcohol as an obstetrical analgesic. Am J Obstet Gynecol 61:676, 1951.
176. Fuchs F, Fuchs AR, Poblete VF Jr, Risk A: Effect of alcohol on threatened premature labor. Am J Obstet Gynecol 99:627–637, 1967.
177. Zlatnik FJ, Fuchs F: A controlled study of ethanol in threatened premature labor. Am J Obstet Gynecol 142:610–612, 1972.
178. Waltman R, Iniquez F, Iniquez ES: Placental transfer of ethanol and its elimination at term. Obstet Gynecol 40:180–185, 1972.
179. Cook LN, Shott RJ, Andrews BF: Acute transplacental ethanol intoxication. Am J Dis Child 129:1075–1076, 1975.
180. Kim SS, Hodgkinson R: Acute ethanol intoxication and its probable effect on a full-term neonate. Anesth Analg Curr Res 55:602–603, 1976.

181. Hollstedt C, Olsson O, Rydberg U: The effect of alcohol on the developing organism: Genetical, teratological and physiological aspects. Med Biol 55:1–14, 1977.
182. Caritis SN, Edelstone DI, Mueller-Heubach E: Pharmacologic inhibition of preterm labor. Am J Obstet Gynecol 133:557, 1979.
183. Fuchs F, Fuchs AR, Lauersen NH, Zervoudakis IA: Treatment of preterm labor with ethanol. Danish Med Bull 26:123–124, 1979.
184. Spearing G: Alcohol, indomethacin, and salbutamol. Obstet Gynecol 53:171–174, 1979.
185. Zervoudakis IA, Krauss A, Fuchs F, Wilson KH: Infants of mothers treated with ethanol for premature labor. Am J Obstet Gynecol 137:713, 1980.
186. Niebyl JR, Johnson JWC: Inhibition of preterm labor. Clin Obstet Gynecol 23:115–126, 1980.
187. Fuchs AR, Fuchs F: Ethanol for prevention of preterm birth. Sem Perinatol 5:236–251, 1981.
188. Lauersen NH, Wilson KH, Fuchs FF: The inhibitory effects of ethanol on oxytocin-induced labor at term. J Reprod Med 26:547–550, 1981.
189. Anderson K: Pharmacological inhibition of uterine activity. Acta Obstet Gynecol Scand (Suppl) 108:17–23, 1982.
190. Huddleston JF: Preterm labor. Clin Obstet Gynecol 25:123–136, 1982.
191. Caritis SN, Carson D, Greebon D, McCormick M, Edelstone DI, Mueller-Heuback E: A comparison of terbutaline and ethanol in treatment of preterm labor. Am J Obstet Gynecol 142:183–190, 1982.
192. Fuchs AR, Husslein P, Sumulong L, Micha JP, Dawood MY, Fuchs F: Plasma levels of oxytocin and 13,14-dihydro-15-keto prostaglandin F2 alpha in preterm labor and the effect of ethanol and ritodrine. Am J Obstet Gynecol 144:752–759, 1982.
193. Souney PF, Kaul AF, Osathanondh R: Pharmacology of preterm labor. Clin Pharmacol 2:29–44, 1983.
194. Weiner N: Norepinephrine, epinephrine, and the sympathomimetic amines. In Gilman AG, Goodman LS, Gilman A (eds): "The Pharmacological Basis of Therapeutics." 6th Ed. New York: Macmillan, 1980, pp 138–175.
195. Sisenwein FE, Tejani NA, Boxer HS, DiGiuseppe R: Effects of maternal ethanol infusion during pregnancy on the growth and development of children at four to seven years of age. Am J Obstet Gynecol 147:52, 1983.
196. Peden VH, Sammon TJ, Downey DA: Intravenously induced infantile intoxication with ethanol. Fetal Neonatal Med 83:490–493, 1973.
197. Niven RG: Alcoholism—A problem in perspective. J Am Med Assoc 252:1912–1914, 1984.
198. Council on Scientific Affairs: Fetal effects of maternal alcoholic use. J Am Med Assoc 249:2517–2521, 1984.

3

Neuronal and Synaptic Organization of the Motor Nuclei of Mammalian Thalamus

Kristy Kultas-Ilinsky and Igor A. Ilinsky

The part of the thalamus that receives projections from basal ganglia and cerebellum and projects further to the neocortex is believed to be an integrative center of the central motor control system. This review summarizes the currently available data on the light and electron microscopy of the motor thalamic nuclei in different species. The discussion is focused on the ventral anterior (VA), ventral medial (VM), and ventral lateral (VL) nuclei of the cat. The relevant data from rat and monkey when available are treated in comparative perspective. We discuss 1) cytological features and relationships of the two major cell types—thalamocortical projection neurons and local circuit neurons in individual subdivisions of the motor thalamus, and 2) mode of termination of cortical, basal ganglia, and cerebellar projections on these two cell types. Although a number of anatomical and physiological properties of the cells in the motor thalamus need to be clarified, it is apparent that there are significant differences in synaptic organization between the VL (the major recipient of the cerebellar projections) and VA and VM (the major projection zones of basal ganglia efferents). It is also apparent that synaptic organization of the motor thalamus changes dramatically in the course of evolutionary specialization. These changes are expressed in a progressive increase of complexity of synaptic arrangements with involvement of the processes of local circuit neurons.

From the Department of Anatomy, The University of Iowa College of Medicine, Iowa City, Iowa 52242, USA.

Current Topics in Research on Synapses, Volume 3, pages 77–145 © 1986 Alan R. Liss, Inc.

1 INTRODUCTION

"The thalamus has not received the same degree of attention as the cerebral cortex and we know very little about its integrative capacities in any of the pathways traversing it." This statement about the thalamus in general by E.G. Jones [1] is even more true if applied to the part of the thalamus directly involved in motor control. Neuroanatomy of this region has been studied relatively little in comparison with other thalamic nuclear groups such as the somatosensory, visual and auditory. Nonetheless, recent findings indicate that many features of neuronal and synaptic relationships observed in the motor thalamus are not represented in other thalamic nuclei. In addition, interspecies differences in the synaptic organization of the motor nuclei appear to be more pronounced than in other thalamic regions. In the present review we intend to summarize the data available on the synaptic organization of the motor thalamus and identify those areas in need of further exploration.

Several studies providing the basic knowledge of neuronal and synaptic organization of the motor thalamus became available in the late 1960s and early 1970s [2–11]. The main limitation of these studies was that the findings were not related to individual cytoarchitectural entities or to the principal domains of specific afferent projection systems within this region. Rather, the area was treated as a whole, thus implying its structural and functional homogeneity. This is understandable, considering the limited knowledge on the topography of afferent inputs to the region at the time. However, in view of the light microscope hodological data accumulated during the last decade, such an approach can no longer be justified. This is because individual cytoarchitectural subdivisions within the motor thalamus differ in regard to their afferent and efferent connections [12–40], differences that should be reflected in the ultrastructure and organization of intrinsic neuronal circuitry.

In order to facilitate discussions of the synaptology of this region, a brief review of the connectional relationships of the motor-related thalamic nuclei and relevant comments on their nomenclature are outlined at the beginning.

2 DEFINITION OF THE MOTOR THALAMUS AND ITS NUCLEAR SUBDIVISIONS

The motor thalamus has been traditionally recognized as the thalamic region that receives projections from the cerebellum and basal ganglia and in turn has direct connections with the motor and premotor cortices. In nonprimates three cytoarchitectural subdivisions fall into this category: ventral anterior (VA), ventral lateral (VL), and ventral medial (VM) thalamic nuclei. In the primate thalamus further cytoarchitectonic distinctions have been recognized [41–44]. In Olszewski's classification of the monkey thalamus [45] the VA is divided into two subnuclei: medial magnocellular (VAmc) and lateral parvocellular (VA proper). The VL in turn consists of a number of subdivisions - pars oralis (VLo), pars medialis (VLm), and pars caudalis (VLc). Moreover, the "area X" and pars oralis of the ventral posterior lateral nucleus (VPLo) are also a part of the motor thalamus in primates, since they receive a massive input from deep cerebellar nuclei [14]. In all species the cytoarchitectural boundaries of the whole complex are quite distinct from those of adjacent nuclear groups, whereas within the complex itself delineation of individual subdivisions has posed certain difficulties. As acknowledged by several authors [1,14,15,26, 29,38,46], the latter fact has led to nomenclature confusions and consequent discrepancies in interpretation of experimental results. The situation becomes even more complicated when different species are compared. Homologies are not always straightforward and additional data are necessary for any further progress in this area. Most of the available data about the synaptic organization of the motor thalamus, concerning both anatomical and electrophysiological aspects, are derived from studies in the cat. The following discussion, therefore, is centered on the data obtained from this species. The data from other species, when available, are considered in comparative terms.

3 TOPOGRAPHY OF SUBCORTICAL PROJECTIONS TO THE MOTOR THALAMUS AND THEIR RELATIONSHIP TO THE CYTOARCHITECTURAL BOUNDARIES OF INDIVIDUAL SUBDIVISIONS

The recent advances in pathway tracing with modern neuroanatomical techniques make it possible to reevaluate the cytoarchitectural subdivisions in the motor thalamus by relating them to the projection zones of subcortical afferents. This subject has been discussed by Ilinsky and Kultas-Ilinsky [29] in relation to the cat thalamus, and by Asanuma et al. [15] in relation to the monkey thalamus. In this review we will follow the delineations of individual thalamic subdivisions as suggested in the above communications.

3.1 Distribution of Basal Ganglia and Cerebellar Afferents

Using the pathway tracing data currently available, the boundaries of the VA in the cat can be established based on the extent of the pallidal projection zone [29]. In this way the posterior boundary of the VA with the VL can be determined accurately regardless of the fact that it is not obvious on purely cytoarchitectural grounds. Similarly the nigrothalamic projection zone can be used for delineation of the VM, especially its lateral boundary with the VL [28,35]. Finally, delineation of the VL can be based on the extent of the projections from the dentate nucleus of the cerebellum [29]. As the light microscope data indicate, the dentate projection zone in the cat does not occupy the whole mediolateral and anteroposterior extent

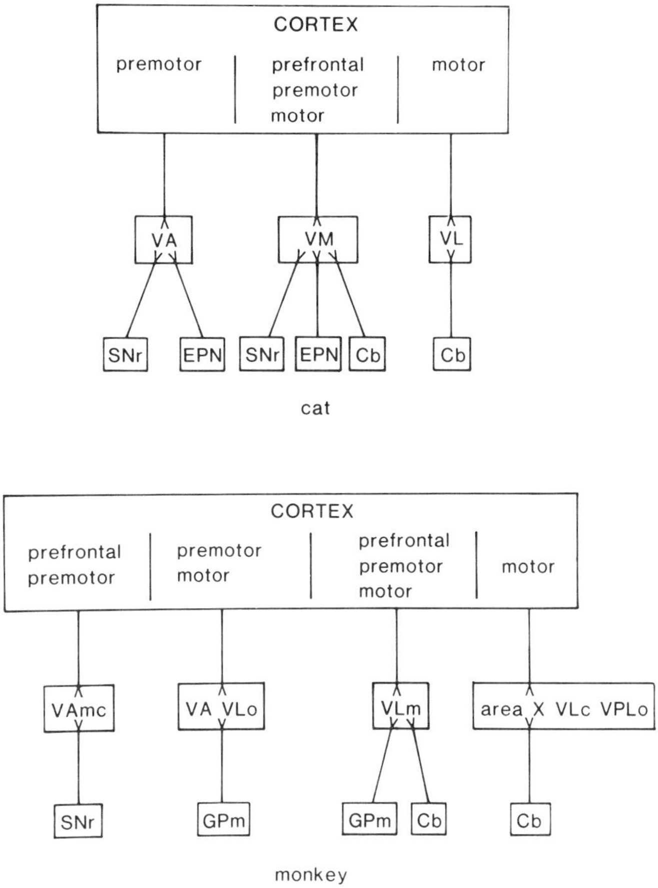

Fig. 1. Summary diagram of major connections of nuclear subdivisions of the motor thalamus in the cat and monkey. For references see text (Section 3).

of the conventional VL, as delineated in available atlases [47–49], whereas the lateroposterior region receives considerable spinothalamic input [16,50]. Comparison of published data on the topography of the cerebello- and spinothalamic projections suggests that there is no significant overlap, if any, between the two systems in the cat VL. Thus, one may suggest that the most lateroposterior region of the cat VL, as delineated in available atlases, should be considered as a separate subdivision.

Distribution of subcortial and cortical projections to the subdivisions of the cat motor thalamus is summarized in Figure 1. In the cat the VA is a recipient of basal ganglia afferents from the pars reticularis of substantia nigra (SNr) and entopeduncular nucleus (EPN), and the VL (excluding its most lateroposterior part) is the recipient of cerebellar afferents (Cb) from the dentate nucleus. On the other hand, the VM, which receives nigral projections throughout its whole extent, is also a recipient of projections from EPN in its anterolateral region and those from Cb in its posterolateral region. The data available on the topographical distribution of cerebellar projections from the nuclei other than dentate, although somewhat controversial, indicate that the projections from nucleus interpositus, for the most part, overlap with those from the dentate in the VL and also probably reach the VA [13,39]. The fastigial input is primarily directed to the VM and, to a lesser extent, to the VL and the VA [12,39]. Nevertheless, additional studies are needed to determine the precise topography of the latter projection systems in this species.

It should be mentioned here that in rodents the situation is different from that in the cat. Although the data in the rat, for example, are difficult to compare, since the nomenclature of thalamic nuclei varies greatly in different studies, one gets the impression that the degree of overlap of the subcortical inputs to the motor thalamus in this species is much higher than in the cat [19–21,23–25,27,51].

In primates, on the other hand, subcortical projections to the motor thalamus are entirely segregated (Fig. 1). Thus, the nigral projection zone (SNr) is confined to the VAmc [18,30,31], pallidal afferents (GPm) are distributed to the VA, VLo, and VLm [22,30,34], and the cerebellar input (Cb) is targeted to area X, VLc, and VPLo [14,32,38,52]. There are some indications that the cerebellar input also reaches VLm (Ilinsky and Kultas-Ilinsky, unpublished). However, pallidal and cerebellar afferents have specific topographical locations within the VLm, and thus both systems also seem to be segregated within the nucleus.

3.2 Thalamocortical and Corticothalamic Projections

Reciprocal connections between the cortex and thalamus are well known and the motor-related thalamic region is not an exception in this respect. Nevertheless, a reevaluation of cortical targets of individual nuclei within the motor thalamus should be done, using the available data on topographical distribution of different subcortical afferent systems. The data currently available indicate that the cerebellar territory of the thalamus (VL in the cat, "cell-sparse zone" in the monkey, which includes area X, VLc, and VPLo) projects preferentially to the primary motor cortex [14,26,40,53,54], as indicated in Figure 1. Projections from the basal ganglia territory of the thalamus are more complex and differ in the two species. Thus, in the cat, VA and VM both project to the premotor and prefrontal cortices [55,56]. Additionally, each individual nucleus has a number of other cortical targets [26,55,57–59]. In the monkey, segregated nigral and pallidal territories in the thalamus have their preferential cortical targets in prefrontal and premotor cortices, respectively, and only a minor overlap of the two systems seems to exist at the cortical level [31,60].

When the exact topography of corticothalamic projections related to major subcorticothalamic inputs is finalized, the classification of the motor thalamic nuclei can be further refined. Relevant to the purposes of this review is the fact that all motor thalamic nuclei receive cortical afferents from the areas they project to [1,61], and this input overlaps with one or several subcortical inputs in each subdivision. Convergence of various afferent inputs in the same thalamic nuclei provides grounds for integration of different activities at the thalamic level before they reach the neocortex. Based on the data discussed above, it appears that there are more possibilities for interaction of different projection systems in the motor thalamus of the rat and cat than in the monkey. Moreover, within the cat motor thalamus, VM is the nucleus where most convergence could occur.

3.3 Do Several Subcortical Afferents Converge on the Same Neurons?

Electrophysiological studies in the rat have demonstrated convergence of cerebellar and nigral inputs on the VM cells [62–65]. In the cat VM, however, no convergence of cerebellar and nigral inputs has been detected [66,67]. In other electrophysiological studies in the cat [66–70] no convergence has been found for other combinations of subcortical afferents despite the obvious overlap of some of the projection systems demonstrated in light microscope studies (for example, projections from two basal ganglia sources). This absence of convergence means that, even in the areas of overlap, the subcortical inputs are nevertheless segregated at the level of individual neurons. This suggests the existence in the same area of different subpopulations of thalamocortical projection neurons, each receiving specific subcortical input. However, this needs to be confirmed by further electrophysiological experiments specifically aimed at exploring the areas of overlap of different projection systems demonstrated in recent anatomical studies [26,28,29]. In the monkey, electrophysiological data are only available for the relationships of pallidal and cerebellar inputs [71,72]. No convergence of these two afferent systems on individual neurons was found; this is in complete agreement with the light microscope hodological data demonstrating the segregation of these pathways to different thalamic subdivisions.

The species variations in the topographical relationships of afferent systems to the motor thalamus imply that the organizational principle of the motor control pathways at the thalamic level varies with the level of evolutionary specialization. The trend appears to be towards the complete segregation of different subcortico-thalamo-cortical pathways.

3.4 Other Possible Afferents

So far we have discussed the major, well-documented afferent projections to the motor thalamus. These, however, do not exhaust the list of potential afferent inputs to the area. One of the additional systems that has been suggested is the reticular nucleus of the thalamus (Rt). This nucleus is considered to provide inhibitory input to all major thalamic nuclei and thus regulate the discharge pattern of thalamic neurons (for recent review see Steriade and Deschênes [73]). This connection was first suggested by Scheibel and Scheibel [74], based on their observations of Golgi-impregnated cells of Rt. They followed the Rt axons to different thalamic nuclei and reported the presence of terminal arborizations in some of them. Later, using anterograde and retrograde tracers, Jones [75] demonstrated Rt projections to a number of thalamic nuclei such as the somatosensory, intralaminar, geniculate, and lateroposterior group of the cat and monkey. Recently, Herkenham and Gerfen [76], using anterograde tracers, have demonstrated Rt connections to the VL and lateral VM in the rat. Projections from the Rt to the cat motor nuclei have also been suggested in a retrograde tracing study of Steriade et al. [77], who demonstrated massive projections from all parts of the Rt to the intralaminar nuclei and only a sparse projection to the VL.

In summary, it appears that the evidence for Rt projections to the motor thalamus is far from convincing, particularly in the cat and monkey. Furthermore, the above data obtained with retrograde tracers have to be treated with caution, since such tracers can be picked up by damaged axons of the fiber systems passing through the area and thus cause false-positive results. For example, the Rt axons destined for the intralaminar nuclei travel through the VA and VL [74] and can be responsible for labeling of the Rt cells when damaged during injection into these nuclei. It has been suggested that the motor nuclei of the thalamus (VA, VM), receiving massive inhibitory input from extrathalamic sources, may lack similar input from the reticular nucleus [78]. This is discussed further in Section 5.2.5.

In the recent literature several reports mention projections to the motor thalamus from the deep layers of the superior colliculus and parabrachial nucleus. The superior colliculus projection to the VA in the Rhesus monkey is well documented and appears to be limited to a small region in the medial part of the VAmc adjacent to the internal medullary lamina [79]. In the rat and cat, however, the anatomical evidence for tectal and parabrachial connections with the motor nuclei of the thalamus is meager and their topography is not known [27,56]. Clearly, further studies are needed to determine the extent and topography of these connections if their existence is proven. Finally, several electrophysiological studies have postulated a direct excitatory pathway to the motor thalamic nuclei from the brain stem reticular formation [65,80,81]. However, no anatomical proof has been forthcoming. On the contrary, the studies that specifically addressed this question, by applying anterograde transport of tritiated amino acids, demonstrated very heavy input from the brainstem reticular formation to the intralaminar nuclei of the thalamus, but none to the adjacent motor nuclei [82].

4 CELL TYPES IN THE MOTOR THALAMUS

There are few descriptive studies dealing with cytological features of nerve cells in the motor thalamus based on the Golgi impregnation technique. One of these described the VA neurons in young animals [11]. The other two investigations described the types of neurons in the VL and VM [7] and VA and VL [9] of adult cats. In neither of these publications was any distinction made between the individual nuclei, thereby implying that no differences were observed. The studies agree that in the motor thalamus there are two major classes of neurons: thalamocortical relay or projection neurons (TCPN), and interneurons or local-circuit neurons (LCN). Each of these classes can be further subdivided into several subcategories.

4.1 Thalamocortical Projection Neurons (TCPN)

4.1.1 Light microscope features of TCPN. Somata of TCPN have either a multipolar or a fusiform shape, and on the basis of the dendritic branching pattern two classes of these cells have been recognized [7,9]. According to these studies primary dendrites of cells with a "tufted" branching pattern generate numerous secondary dendrites at the first branching site; secondary branches in turn give off a few tertiary dendrites. Another type of TCPN ("radiating") is characterized by a more regular branching pattern, a greater number of primary dendrites, and a larger dendritic field compared to the tufted type. Primary dendrites of this cell type give off a couple of short secondary dendrites, which in turn generate numerous long tertiary dendrites.

Additional proof that these cells are TCPN is provided by studies using retrograde HRP labeling of thalamic cells from the pericruciate and proreal cortices [83]. It has not been possible in the cat thalamus, unlike in other species and brain regions [84], to obtain Golgi-type staining of thalamic cells in retrograde labeling experiments with HRP. Nevertheless, in some instances, neuronal processes have been filled with HRP granules

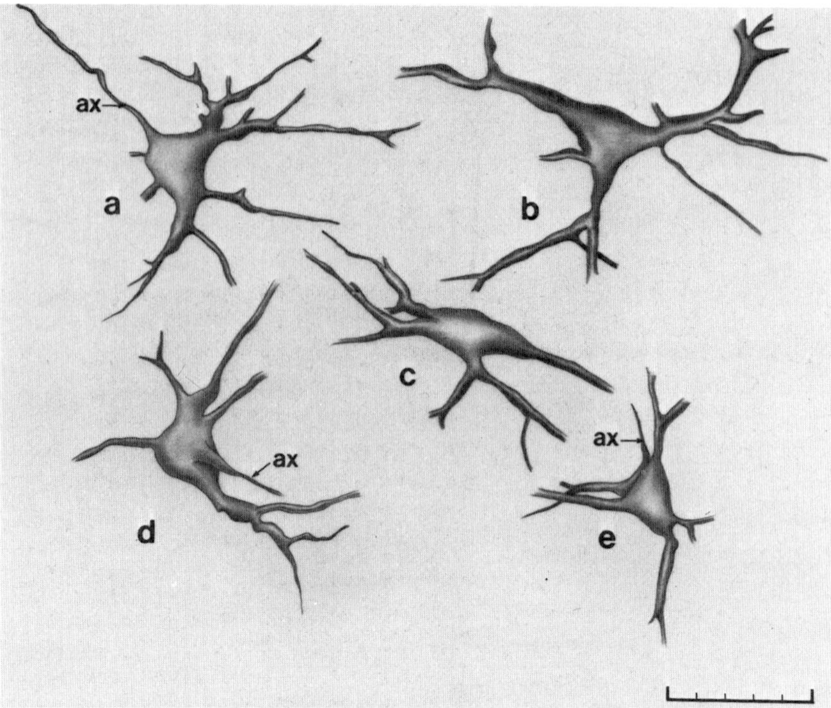

Fig. 2. Camera lucida drawings of a representative sample of HRP-filled cells (TCPN) in the cat VA following injections in the precruciate and proreal gyri of the cortex. Note variations in the size and shape of perikarya of TCPN (a–e), in length and width of primary and secondary dendrites, and in dendritic branching patterns. Ax, axons; scale = 50 μm.

up to the second branching site (Figs. 2–4). This allows the features of labeled cells to be compared with those identified as TCPN in Golgi-impregnated preparations (Fig. 5) of the same nuclei. Analysis of such data reveals remarkable similarities of neuronal features in both types of preparations, thus confirming the identification of these cells as TCPN.

In our Golgi impregnated preparations of the cat motor thalamus we found categorization of the TCPN into subtypes to be difficult [85]. Typical examples of the two types of TCPN (tufted and radiating) described in earlier studies are rarely encountered and the great majority of cells exhibit mixed dendritic arborization patterns. The same impression is gained from HRP-labeled cells. In the same cell some primary dendrites can be short and give rise to tufts of secondary branches, whereas other primary dendrites are long (up to 40 μm) and divide dichotomically, and secondary dendrites give rise to 2–6 tertiary dendrites. In some instances the cells have thick primary dendrites that give off a number of much

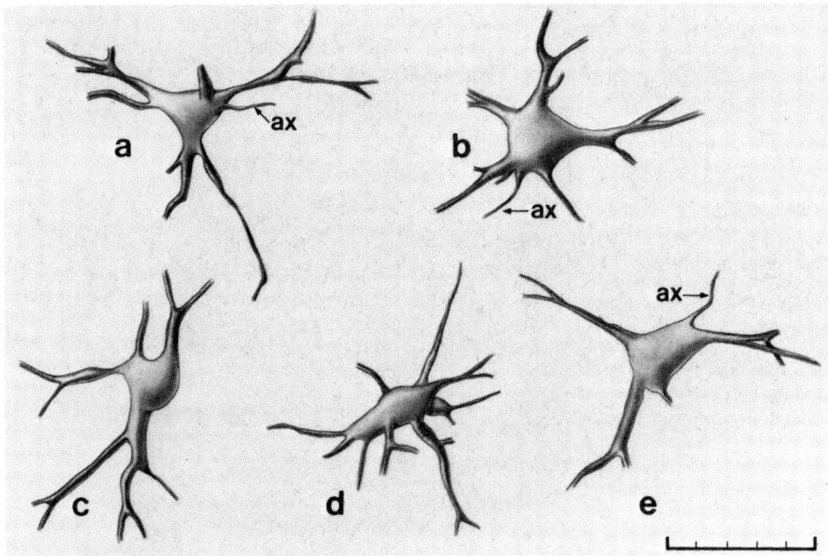

Fig. 3. Camera lucida drawings of a representative sample of HRP-filled cells (TCPN) in the cat VM following injections in the precruciate and proreal gyri of the cortex. Note the smaller size of perikarya of TCPN (a–e) compared to those in the VA and the less variable dendritic branching pattern. Ax, axons; scale = 50 μm.

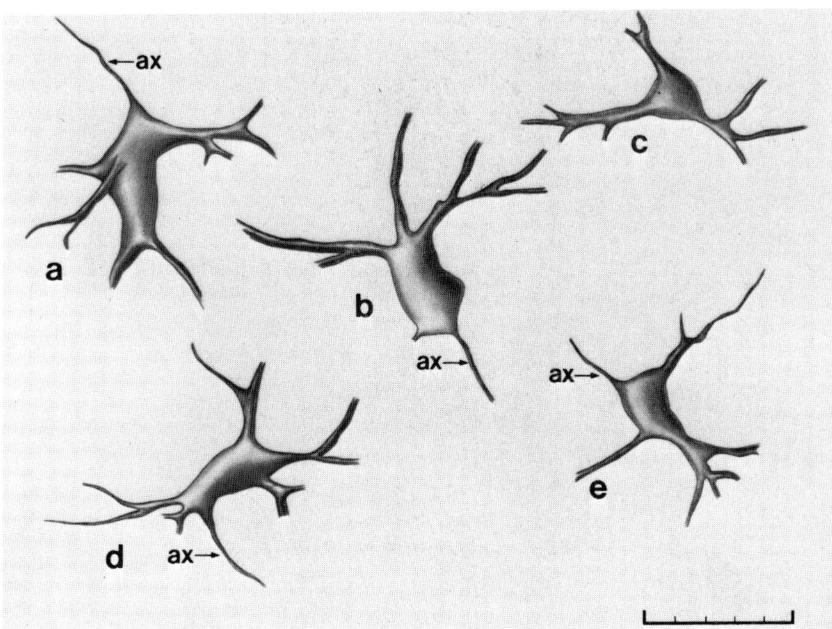

Fig. 4. Camera lucida drawings of HRP-filled cells (TCPN) in the cat VL following injections in the lateral parts of pre- and postcruciate gyri of the cortex. Note the wider range of sizes of TCPN somata (a–e) compared to those in the VM, and the presence of both tufted and radiating dendritic branching patterns in the same cells (a,b,e). Ax, axons, scale = 50 μm.

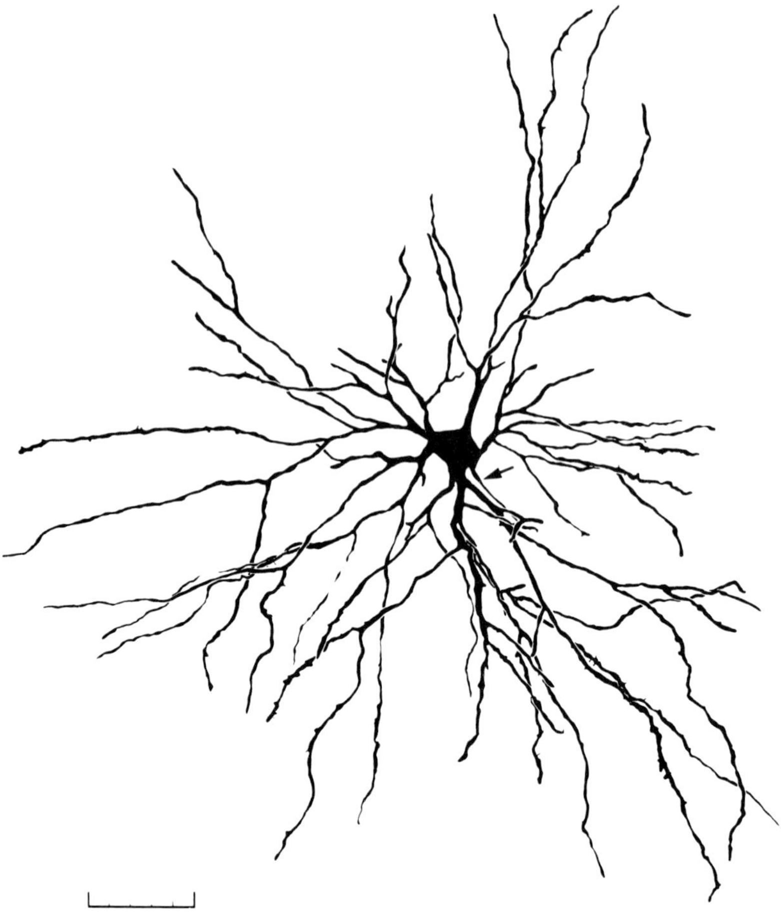

Fig. 5. An example of a Golgi-impregnated neuron (TCPN) in the cat VM. Arrow points to the initial part of an axon. Note the variations in the length and width of primary and secondary dendrites. Camera lucida drawing, zinc chromate modification of the Golgi technique. Scale = 50 μm. From Al-Hussain and Kultas-Ilinsky [85].

thinner side branches. It should be stressed that the width of different-order dendritic branches is quite variable. For instance, some of the primary dendrites can be of about the same width as secondary or even tertiary branches of the same cell [85].

According to our preliminary data the differences between the three nuclei primarily concern the size of TCPN. The results of measurements of the somata of VM cells are presented in Table I. The average diameter of TCPN in the VM is about 22 μm. This appears to be slightly smaller

TABLE I. Dimensions and ratio of HRP-positive and HRP-negative cells in the VM following injections in precruciate and proreal gyri of the cat cortex

Exp. animal	N	HRP-positive cells (μm) Dm	Dl	Ds	N	HRP-negative cells (μm) Dm	Dl	Ds	Ratio HRP+ cells/ HRP− cells
C71	46	21.5	24	18	20	13.2	16.1	10.3	3/1
SD		1.7	5.58	1.7		1.27	2.4	1.48	
C83	30	23	25.5	20.5	18	13.5	16.32	10.8	3/1
SD		1.34	1.78	2.55		1.3	2.82	1.41	
Total & mean, 2 cats	76	22.25	24.7	19.7	38	13.3	16.2	10.5	3/1

N, number of cells measured; Dl, mean long diameter; Ds, mean short diameter; Dm, mean average diameter calculated for each cell as (Dl + Ds)/2. Only cells with nucleolus present in the section plane were measured. Measurements were performed on photomicrographs of 1-μm-thick Epon sections such as shown in Figure 6 with the Bioquant image analysis system.

than the diameters of cells in the VA and VL, which are around 27 μm based on our preliminary data. Moreover, it appears that the cells in the VA exhibit greater variability of sizes and branching patterns than do those in the VL and VM (Figs. 2–4).

It is well known that the branching pattern of dendritic arbors determines the manner in which the afferent information arriving at different-order dendritic branches reaches the soma and influences the spike generation at a trigger zone [86,87]. The features of dendritic arbors of neurons in the motor thalamus, especially the great variability of branching patterns of the dendrites of the same cell, suggest that different mechanisms may be involved in impulse propagation along the tufted and long radiating dendrites of the same neuron. Morphometric studies on dendritic patterns of TCPN in the motor nuclei of the thalamus are currently in progress in our laboratory in order to quantify the general characteristics of these cells. An understanding of the properties of the TCPN dendrites will have to wait until the correlative data between dendritic arborization patterns and the distribution of various afferent inputs along different types of dendrites become available.

Axons of TCPN are readily recognizable in HRP preparations, where they can be followed for some distance (Figs. 2–4). They usually originate from well-defined axon hillocks and at short distances from the soma acquire a lateral course towards the internal capsule. No axon collaterals of these cells ramifying within the nuclei of origin have been identified in our material either in HRP or in Golgi preparations. A similar conclusion was reached by Steriade and Deschênes [73], based on their observations of an electrophysiologically identified TCPN in the VL filled intracellularly with HRP. Likewise in a recently published study by Yamamoto et al. [88] no recurrent axon collaterals were found in HRP-filled cells that were electrophysiologically identified as TCPN. However, the results of these authors were ambivalent in that they also found a few cells with morphological features, similar to those of identified TCPN, that displayed axon collaterals within the confines of parent nuclei. Although the physiological identification of these cells as TCPN was not available, Yamamoto et al. [88] considered these results as indication that the recurrent TCPN axon collaterals do exist.

4.1.2 Fine structure of TCPN. The ultrastructural features of the TCPN have been described in the cat VA and VL by Rinvik and Grofová [9] and in VM by Kultas-Ilinsky et al. [83]. These cells can be recognized in EM preparations by abundant cytoplasm that is rich in organized RER and other organelles. Typical somata of TCPN, identified by the presence of retrogradely transported HRP granules, are seen in Figures 6 and 7. Primary and secondary dendrites of these cells have smooth contours and lack typical spines (Figs. 7,8). Occasionally, however, bulb-like protrusions are seen projecting from their surface. These bulbous protrusions contain whorls of microfilaments and several mitochondria (Fig. 19). They are attached by means of puncta adherentes to adjacent profiles of synaptic boutons and occasionally also receive synaptic contacts (Fig. 19). Additionally, the dendritic membrane is characterized by the presence of small bulges that are usually associated with the postsynaptic part of synaptic contacts. The number and height of such bulges increase significantly on tertiary dendrites (Fig. 9). A few short-stem spines may also be present on tertiary dendrites. However, these never contain a spine apparatus and do not always bear synaptic terminals.

A well-known limitation of ultrastructural studies of nerve tissue is the difficulty in establishing the continuity of different-order branches belonging to the same cell type, since only portions of dendrites are usually seen in thin sections. Therefore, in the majority of ultrastructural studies on the synaptic organization of different brain regions, the diameter of the dendrites observed in the neuropil has been the sole criterion used for determination of the proximity of particular dendritic branches to soma. In some instances far-reaching conclusions have been made based on this type of analysis [89].

From the above description of Golgi-impregnated cells in the motor thalamus it is obvious that size as a criterion is not applicable in this brain region, since a wide overlap of diameters of different-order dendritic branches can be expected. Consequently, we explored the possibility

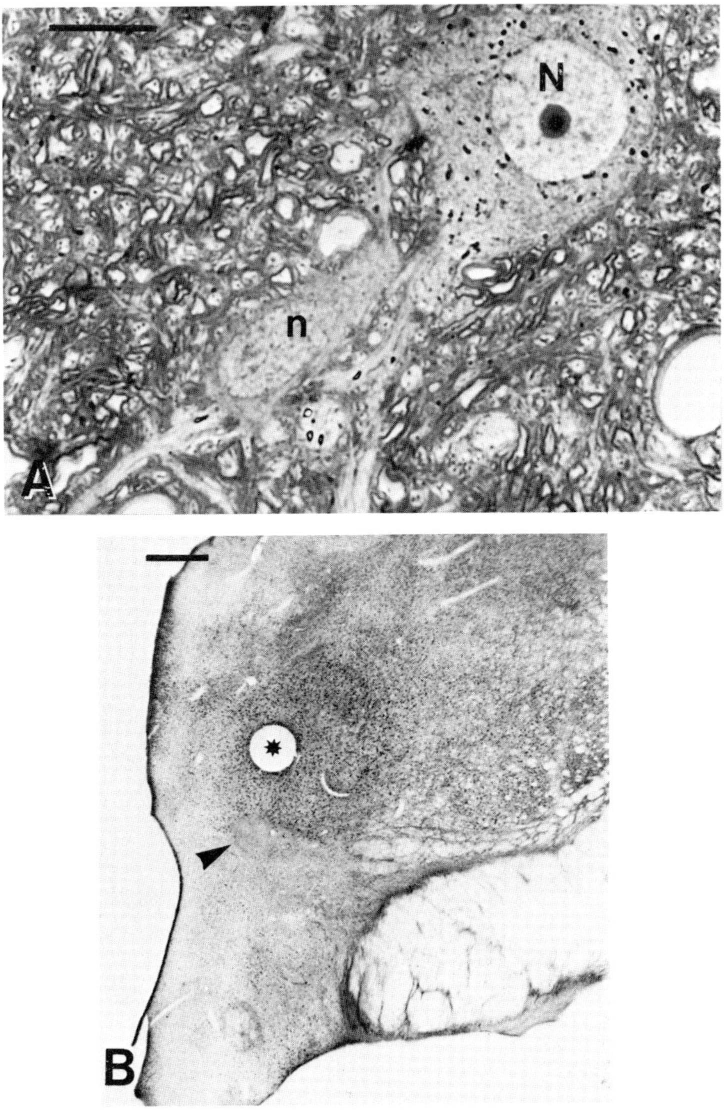

Fig. 6. A. Phase contrast micrograph of a large HRP-labeled cell (N) and a small HRP-negative cell (n) in the VM after cortical injection of HRP (1-μm Epon section, bar = 10 μm). B. Low-power micrograph of a frontal section through the thalamus demonstrating the distribution of retrogradely labeled cells in the motor thalamus after cortical injection of HRP in precrucriate and proreal gyri. Asterisk indicates the position of an EM specimen punched out from the VM and used for analysis of cytological features and sizes of labeled and unlabeled cells. Arrowhead points to the mammillothalamic tract. A 100-μm vibratome section; HRP reaction according to protocol of Malmgren and Olsson [118]. Counterstained for Nissl. Bar = 1 mm.

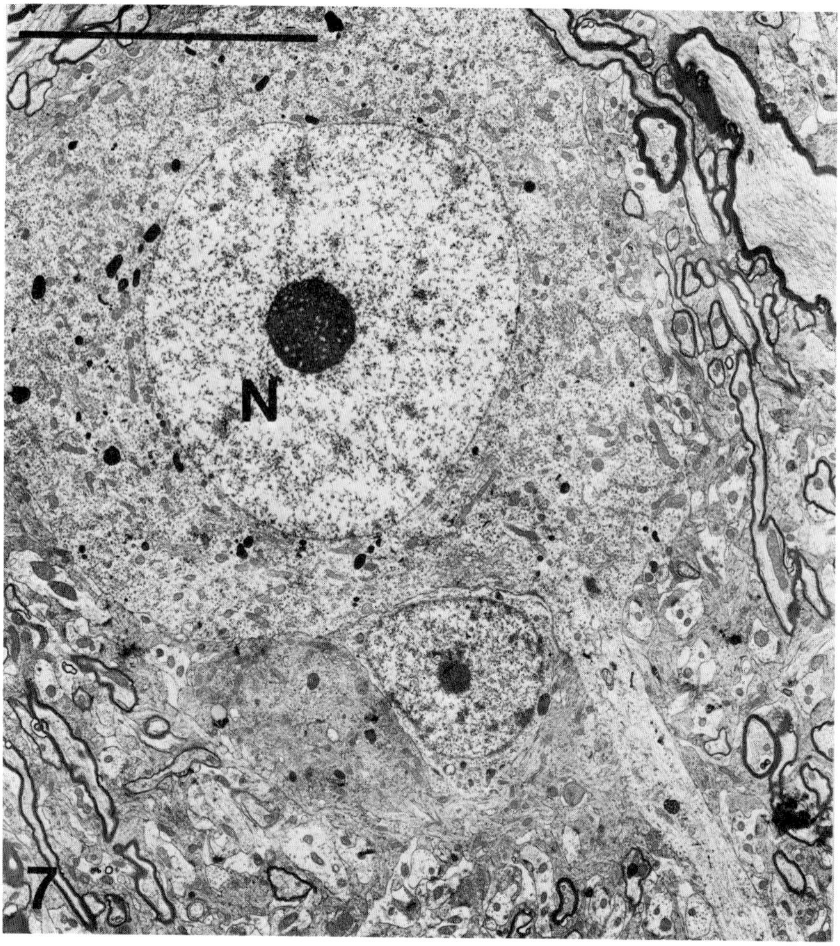

Fig. 7. Electron micrograph of TCPN in the VM containing HRP granules in soma and primary dendrite. N, nucleus. Cortical injection site as described in Figure 3. Bar = 10 μm.

whether ultrastructural features other than diameter can be used for identification of the order of dendrite branches of TCPN. We analyzed examples of the dendrites seen in continuity from the soma to distant parts of tertiary branches in the same sections. The findings indicated that in the motor thalamic nuclei it is possible to identify a set of ultrastructural features specific for different-order dendritic branches of TCPN, and these can be effectively applied in ultrastructural analysis of random neuropil. In particular, the primary dendrites of TCPN in VA, VM, and VL are

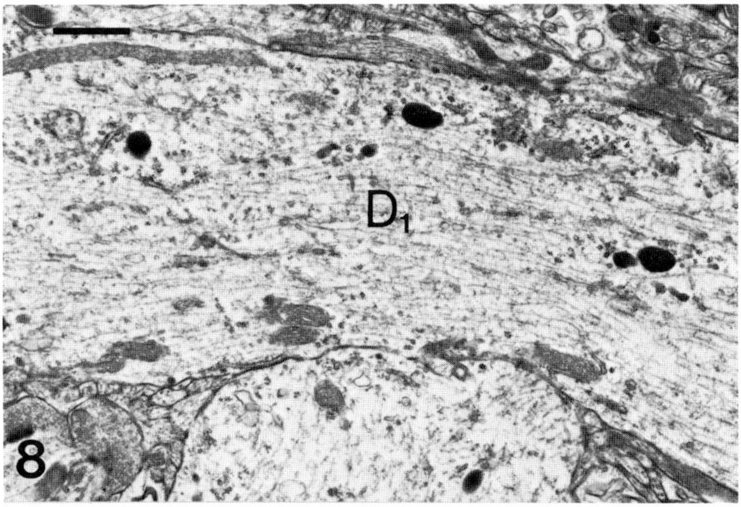

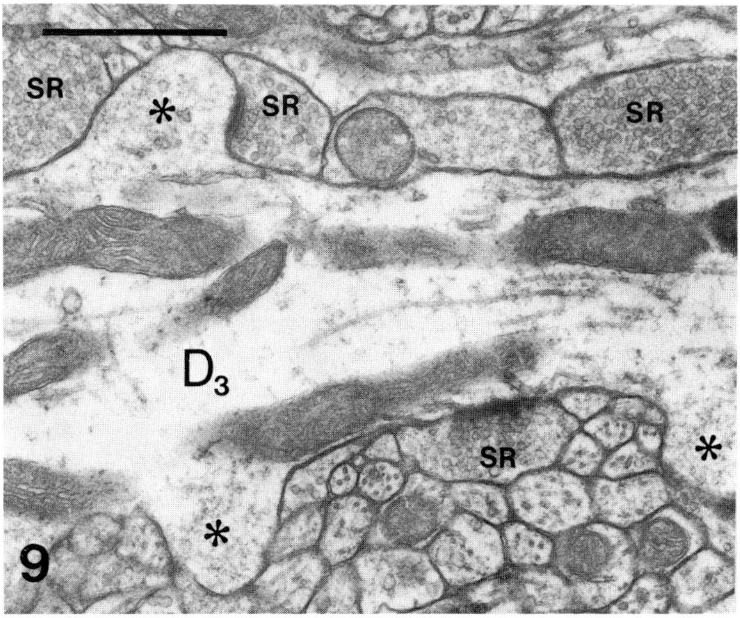

Fig. 8. Ultrastructural features of primary TCPN dendrite (D_1). Note richness in organelles (RER, mitochondria, lysosomes), and high density and regular arrangement of neurotubules. Bar = 1 μm.

Fig. 9. Ultrastructural features of a tertiary TCPN dendrite (D_3). Note the presence of numerous mitochondria, scarcity of neurotubules, and uneven outlines due to bulges (asterisks). SR, small axon terminals containing round synaptic vesicles and forming asymmetrical contacts; two such contacts are seen in the plane of section. Bar = 1 μm.

characterized by a high density of neurotubules that are organized in parallel rows in an orderly fashion (Fig. 8). In between the neurotubules large numbers of polyribosomal rosettes, lysosomes, and mitochondria are present. At the first branching point, accumulation of numerous mitochondria and RER are usually found (Fig. 30), and profiles of Golgi apparatus are occasionally seen. In the secondary dendrites the orderly arrangement of neurotubules is retained, whereas the number of ribosomes and mitochondria is significantly reduced (Fig. 10). Those present show a tendency to be located along the cross-sectional perimeter of the dendrite, immediately beneath the plasma membrane. Interestingly, these same features are displayed by secondary branches regardless of up to threefold differences in width quite often observed between them. Tertiary dendrites are characterized by a rather translucent matrix, the presence of numerous mitochondria, and a remarkably reduced density and irregular arrangement of neurotubules (Fig. 9).

Synaptic coverage of the TCPN membrane is very low on soma and primary dendrites, increasing distally and being the densest on tertiary dendrites. No synaptic contacts have been found on the axon initial segments of the TCPN. Essential differences are found between the three motor nuclei of the thalamus in the density and types of synaptic boutons on proximal and distal parts of the TCPN (see Section 6).

4.2 Local-Circuit Neurons (LCN)

4.2.1 Light microscope features of LCN. The LCNs described in published Golgi studies [7,9,11] were characterized as small cells that give off a few slender, long, and varicose dendrites, with relatively few secondary branches from which protrude numerous spine-like projections. These dendritic features make the LCNs easily distinguishable from the TCPNs (Fig. 11). Two subpopulations of LCNs were also recognized [7,11]. In one type the axon was described as ramifying within the parent dendritic arbor ("small field short axon cell" of Scheibels [11] or "type IIa neuron" of Kiss and Tömböl [7]). In the other type ("large field short axon cell" of Scheibels and "type IIb neuron" of Kiss and Tömböl) the axonal branches were said to reach far beyond the parent cell dendritic field but presumably stayed within the confines of each nucleus. In these studies, however, documentation of axonal arborization of the cells identified as LCNs was not very convincing. The investigators mentioned difficulties in the impregnation of axons of presumed interneurons and only short segments of such processes were demonstrated. In all cases these examples were from the VL. Further, statements on the branching patterns of these axons [7] were mostly based on analogy with similar cells in other thalamic nuclei of the cat, such as the ventrobasal complex, where the existence of Golgi type II cells with axons had been previously demonstrated [90].

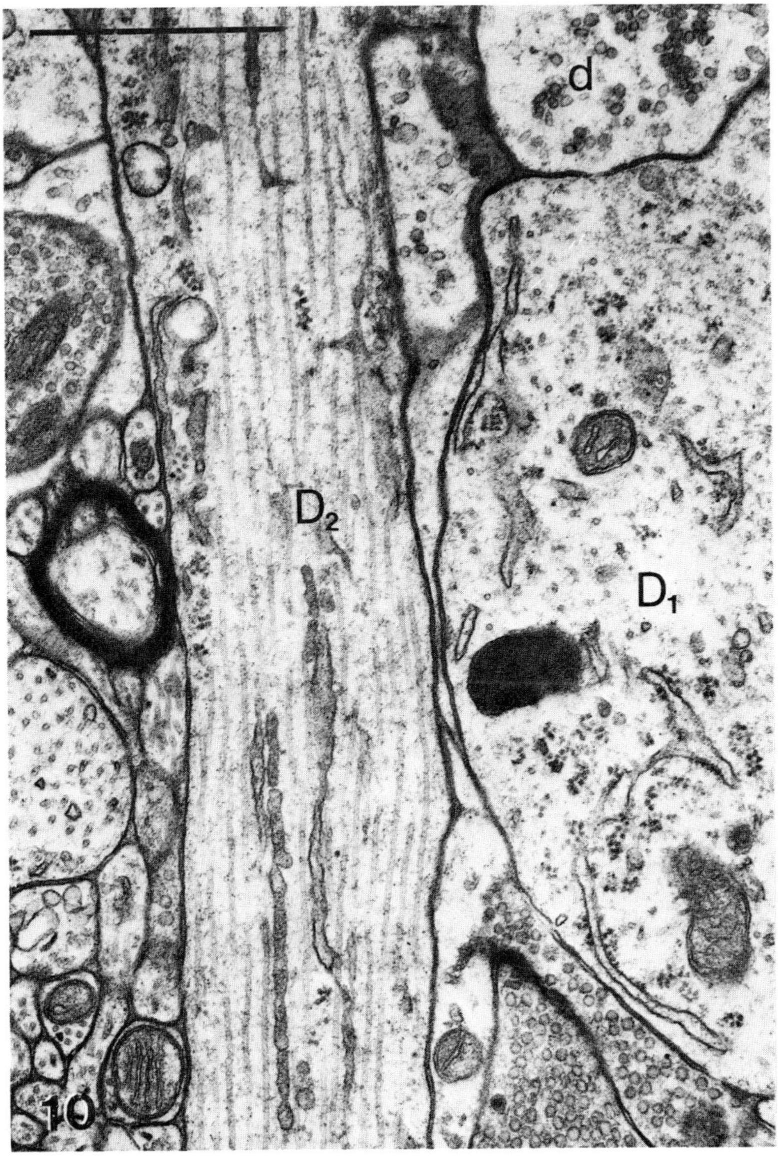

Fig. 10. Ultrastructural features of secondary TCPN dendrite (D_2). Note the absence of mitochondria, high density of neurotubules, and preferential location of RER beneath the plasma membrane. These features can be compared to those of a cross-sectioned primary dendrite (D_1) at right. d, part of a cross-sectioned profile of a vesicle containing dendrite. Bar = 1 μm.

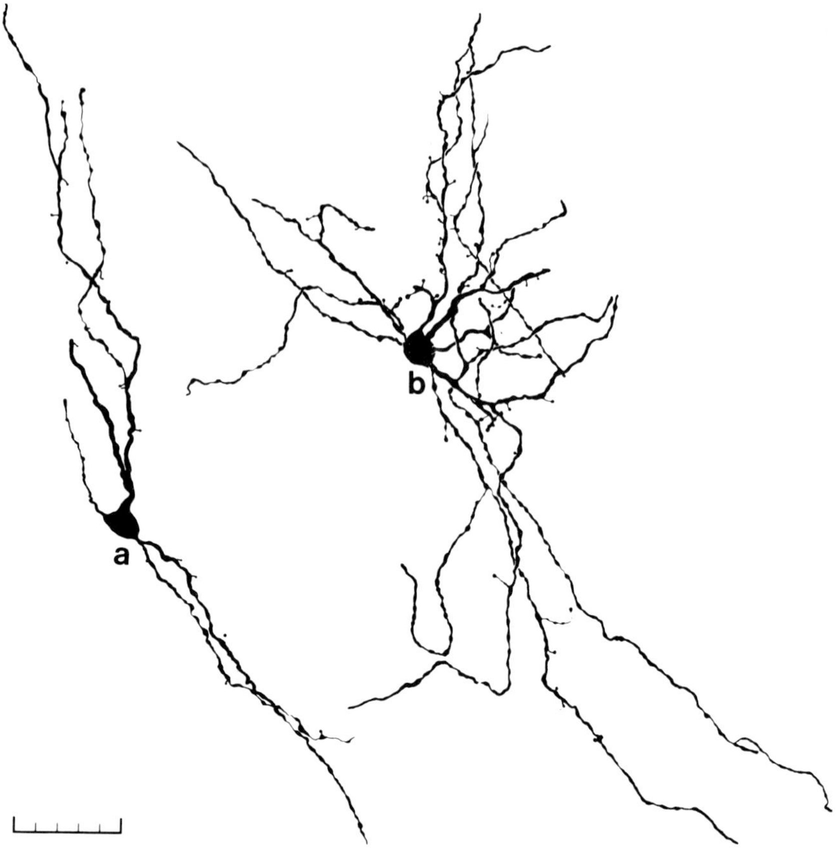

Fig. 11. Examples of Golgi-impregnated small cells (LCNs) in the VA (a) and VL (b). Note varicose outlines of the dendrites and spine-like projections on their surface. Note also a larger dendritic arbor of the cell from the VL (b). Scale 50 μm. (From Al-Hussain and Kultas-Ilinsky, unpublished).

Our observations on Golgi-impregnated material from the cat indicate that the small cells in the VL have much more extensive dendritic arbors than similar cells in the VA and VM (Fig. 11). LCNs with identifiable axons have not yet been seen in either of the motor nuclei studied. However, the secondary dendritic branches arising from the long primary dendrites of LCNs are sometimes very thin and beaded and usually have a very tortuous course. An individual process such as this can easily be interpreted as an axon. However, since these processes originate at different points along primary dendrites, it is likely that they are dendrites. The first electrophysiological study that described LCNs intracellularly filled with HRP in the cat motor thalamus [88] did not solve this problem either. Apparently the authors experienced similar difficulties while trying to differentiate between the dendrites and axons of these cells, since they described "very fine axons with clear varicosity" and additionally "two long axons" as all belonging to the same LCN. Convincing evidence for the existence of the axons of these cells is yet to be obtained. Until then the possibility remains that LCN in the cat motor thalamus, at least in VA and VM, are axonless, as has been suggested for some other thalamic nuclei [91–93].

All available studies agree that most cells identified as interneurons are about half the size of the TCPN, with the exception of a few type IIb LCNs of Kiss and Tömböl [7], the size of which is sometimes close to that of the smallest TCPN. In our experiments, using retrograde labeling of thalamic cells following HRP injections in the cat pericruciate cortex, we consistently found a population of very small cells in the VA, VM, and VL that remained unlabeled. The presence of such cells was not immediately obvious in thick-frozen or vibratome sections routinely used in HRP experiments. However, they were easily identified in 1-μm Epon sections cut from tissue blocks obtained from areas within the motor nuclei containing a large number of retrogradely labeled cells (Fig. 6). In the VM the average length of the short axis of small cells, when measured at the level of the nucleolus, was constant, whereas the length of the long axis was much more variable (Table I), suggesting a cylindrical or fusiform shape of the perikarya. It has been demonstrated recently [78] that in the cat VA, VM, and VL similar small cells are GABAergic, since they show high-intensity immunostaining with antibodies to glutamate decarboxylase (GAD), the major synthetic enzyme of the inhibitory neurotransmitter GABA. It is interesting that this immunocytochemical study also failed to identify the axons of GAD-positive cells.

4.2.2 Fine structure of LCN. At the EM level the small GAD-positive cells are characterized by a relatively large nucleus with deep indentations of the nuclear envelope and a narrow rim of cytoplasm surrounding it [78]. Unlike the cells identified as TCPN, the perikaryal cytoplasm contains little organized RER but mostly scattered ribosomal rosettes and several Golgi profiles (Fig. 12). A characteristic feature of these neurons is the presence of large lobulated lysosomes of moderate electron density (Fig. 13). Since these features are quite different from those of TCPN lysosomes, they can be used as an additional criterion for differentiation between the somata of the LCN and TCPN [78].

Axosomatic synapses on LCN have been demonstrated only in VL but not in the VA and VM nuclei [78]. The synaptic coverage of the LCN dendrites is sparse, especially at proximal levels; distally it is also lower

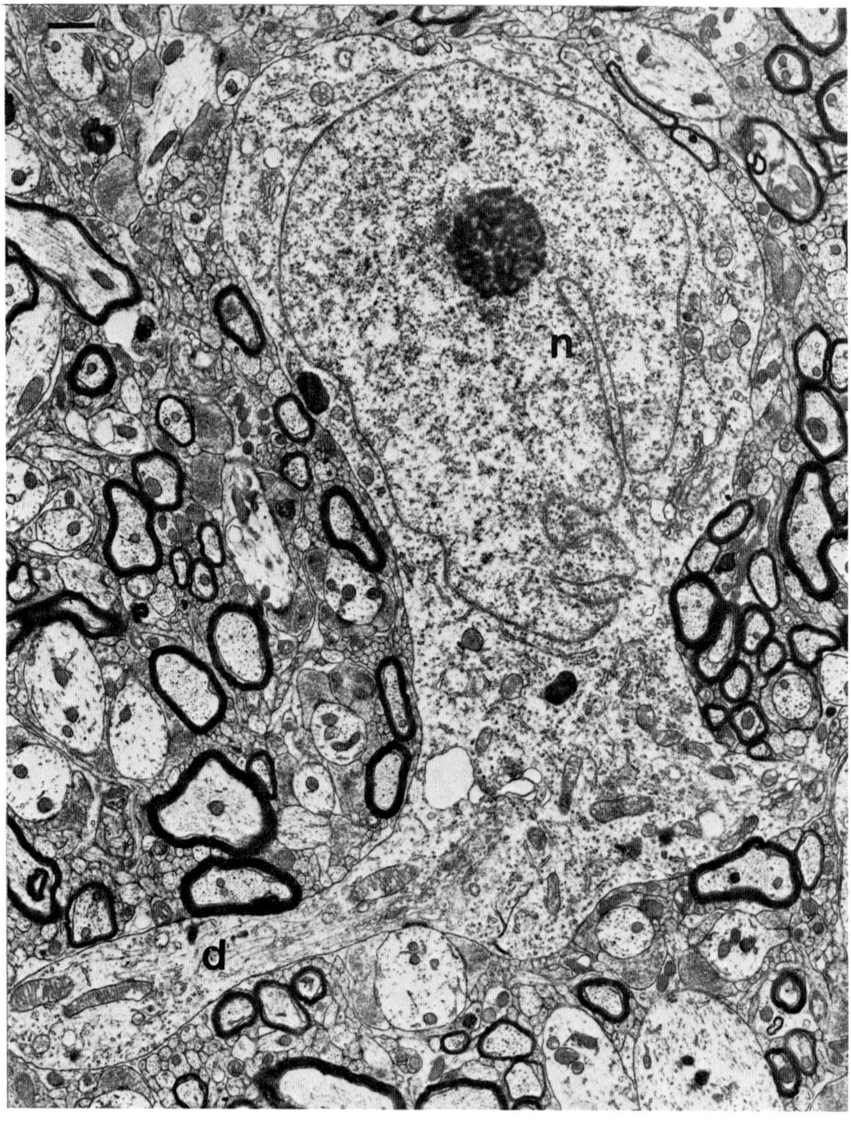

Fig. 12. Electron micrograph of a small cell identified as LCN (n) in the cat VM. Note deep indentations of the nuclear envelope, narrow rim of cytoplasm, and presence of large lysosomes. Serial section analysis reveals that the primary dendrite (d) of this cell contains a group of synaptic vesicles. Note the absence of axosomatic synapses. Bar = 1 μm.

Fig. 13. Electron micrographs illustrating a close apposition of a TCPN (N) and an LCN (n). A. High-magnification electron micrograph of opposing membranes of the two cells shown in B, taken from an adjacent serial section. Note the subsurface location of RER cysterns in the TCPN (N). Arrowhead points to a HRP-positive granule; n, cytoplasm of small HRP-negative cell. Bar = 100 nm. B. Note the presence in the TCPN (N) of HRP granules (arrowheads) retrogradely transported from the injection site in the precruciate and proreal gyri of the cat cortex. Note also the presence of large lobulated lysosomes of moderate electron density (arrow) in the cytoplasm of the LCN (n). Bar = 1 μm.

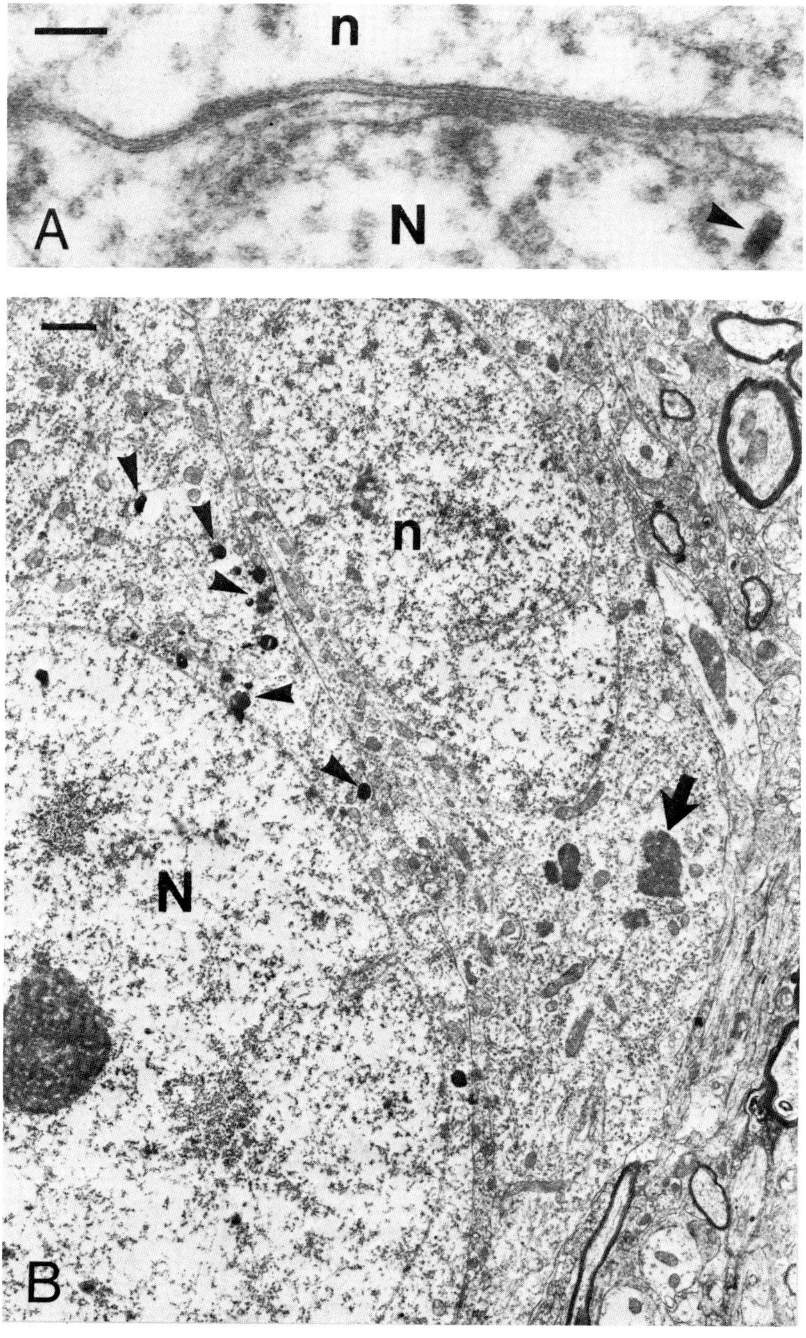

n
A
N
n
N
B

than on TCPN dendrites (Fig. 14). Ultrastructurally, the dendrites of the small cells identified as LCN differ from those of TCPN by the presence of synaptic vesicles. The vesicle-containing dendrites in the motor nuclei of the cat thalamus were first associated with LCN by Rinvik and Grofová [9], who demonstrated such a process in continuity with a neuronal perikaryon. However, these authors noted that the size of the cell from which the vesicle-containing dendrite originated was larger than the average size of the majority of type II neurons. This suggests that the cell described by them may be a representative of a type IIb LCN [7]. An example of a much smaller cell in continuity with a vesicle-containing dendrite observed in the VM is demonstrated in Figure 12.

The proximal dendrites of LCN can be distinguished from the TCPN dendrites by their darker matrix and higher concentration of ribosomes. Our observations show that the vesicles are usually absent in the perikarya of LCN and they are infrequent in the most proximal dendritic shafts. Distally the number of synaptic vesicles increases and they are found in clusters, usually in varicose parts of the dendrites (Fig. 14) as well as within and adjacent to spine-like projections (Fig. 17). Such uneven distribution of synaptic vesicles along the LCN dendrites may explain why examples of LCN somata in continuity with vesicle-containing dendrites are so few. Large numbers of serial sections through these cells are needed to demonstrate such continuity in each case. Another peculiar feature of the LCN dendrites is the dense packing of numerous microtubules in constricted regions and their dispersed arrangement in varicosities (Fig. 14). The vesicle-containing dendrites of LCN are both pre- and postsynaptic to a number of different profiles. The types of synaptic relationships incorporating vesicle-containing dendrites will be described in sections 4.4 and 5.1.

4.3 Other Cell Types in the Motor Thalamus

Evidence of the existence of other cell types in the motor thalamic nuclei is sparse. In several recent neuroanatomical studies it has been shown that a small number of cells in the intralaminar region of VA do not project to the cortex but to the striatum [94–97]. This supports the earlier observations in Golgi studies [7,98], that suggest that some of the large cells of the motor thalamus may project in rostral and caudal directions to brain areas other than the neocortex. Kiss and Tömböl [7] noted that some large cells, whose axons were coursing caudally, differed from those believed to be TCPN, in that they had a fusiform shape with long, straight dendrites emanating from opposite ends of the soma. Recently, additional evidence for caudally projecting cells in the motor nuclei has been obtained in electrophysiological studies in the rat VM [65]. Antidromic spikes were elicited in the VM neurons by stimulation of the mesencephalic reticular formation and superior colliculus. Only 4% of the total population of cells recorded in this study were identified as cells projecting to these caudal structures. This is in agreement with observations of Kiss and Tömböl [7], who noted that fusiform cells of specific morphology were rarely seen in Golgi preparations. In our experiments with retrograde labeling of the cat VM cells from the cortex, the proportion of large labeled cells varied depending on the topography of cortical injections and thalamic sampling sites [83]. It is known that the VM cortical projections in the cat are widespread [56–59], and we did not attempt to inject all VM cortical projection areas. However, injections that involved almost the whole of the pericruciate gyrus resulted in the retrograde labeling of the vast majority of large cells in the lateral VM. In these experiments only one of every 100 large cells counted was unlabeled. The possibility that these unlabeled cells may project to cortical areas other than the pericruciate gyrus cannot be excluded. However, these results may also indicate that, at least in the lateral VM of the cat, caudally projecting neurons may constitute not more than 1% of the total population of large cells.

These data, obtained in different laboratories with different techniques, indicate that a small population of cells differing from the two major types of neurons (TCPN and LCN) may exist in the motor thalamic nuclei. However, additional studies are needed before the actual size of this neuronal population, as well as the cytological characteristics of the cells, can be appreciated in full.

4.4 Relationships Between the TCPN and LCN in the Motor Nuclei

Studies of 1-μm Epon sections as well as EM observations of material obtained from retrograde HRP labeling experiments demonstrate that the somata of both types of cells can be found in close apposition to one another without any intervening structures [Figs. 6A, 13]. Such a relationship is frequently observed in the VA and VM, but only rarely in the VL. Attempts to resolve the membrane specializations between the somata of the adjacent cells (Fig. 13A) have failed. Therefore, the possibility that chemical or electrotonic somatosomatic synapses exist between the LCN and TCPN cannot be confirmed.

The well-established contact between the two types of cells is by means of dendrodendritic synapses [9,78,99] and in a few instances by dendrosomatic [78] synapses, in which the presynaptic part is formed by GAD-positive vesicle-containing dendrites of LCN and the postsynaptic part by TCPN. Synaptic contacts established by the LCN dendrites are symmetrical, with well-pronounced presynaptic dense projections (Figs. 14–16). It has also been noted that these GABAergic dendrodendritic synapses are more numerous in the VL, where they are often found at the bifurcation sites of TCPN dendrites [78]. Two lines of evidence: GAD

ABERYSTWYTH LLYFRGELL C.P.C. ★

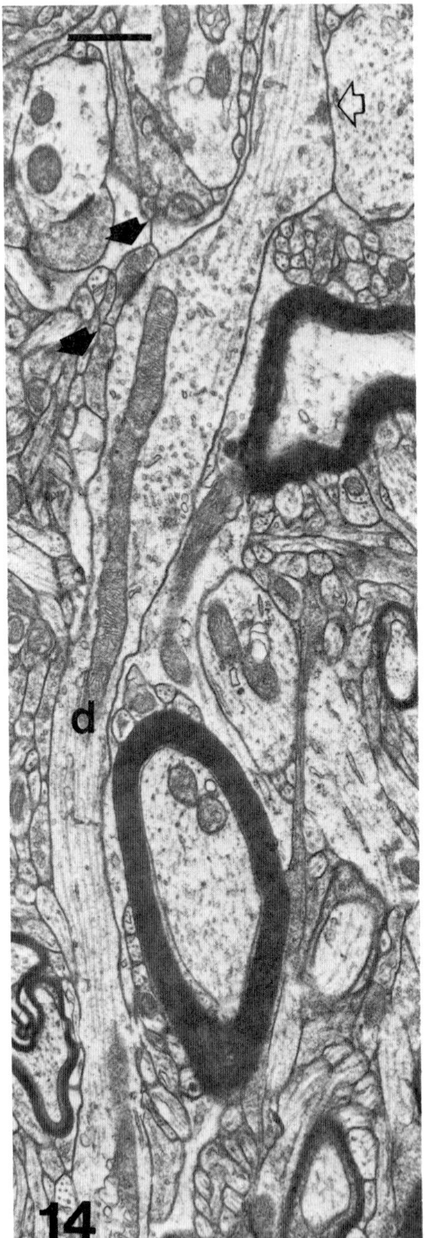
d
14

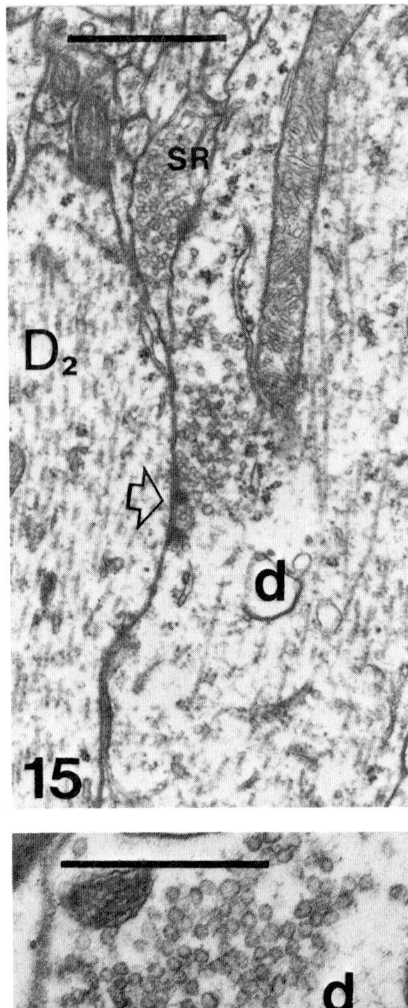
SR
D2
d
15

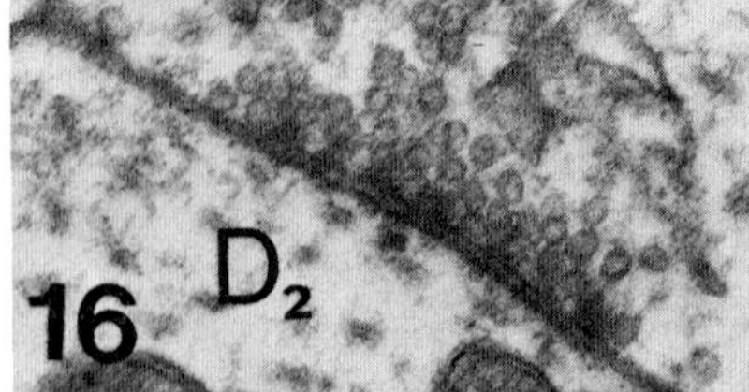
d
D2
16

immunoreactivity of presynaptic dendrites of LCN, and the symmetrical contacts formed by them, strongly favor the inhibitory nature of LCNs in the motor thalamus. Therefore, the influence exerted by these cells on TCPN at dendrodendritic contacts should be inhibitory. However, the overall mechanism of interaction between the two types of cells will remain unclear until the main question about their relationships is resolved. The latter concerns the termination sites of LCN axons on the TCPN, if these axons exist. Needless to say, inhibition provided by an LCN axon terminal at a strategic site of TCPN or inhibition provided by dendrodendritic synapses at distal dendrites will result in quite different effects upon the TCPN firing pattern. Moreover, if both mechanisms are operating, the net effect may be different from that of each individual component.

Another aspect of relationships between the TCPN and LCN requiring determination is the size of the TCPN pool served by one LCN. The numerical ratio of the two cell types (TCPN:LCN) established in experiments with retrograde labeling of TCPN from the pericruciate cortex was found to be 3:1 in the VM (Table I). The ratios of the two cell types in VA and VL are not yet available. In an immunocytochemical study [78] it was noted that the frequency of small GAD-positive cells in the VL was higher than in the VA and VM. It appears, though, that the actual number of TCPNs contacted by one LCN may be significant, considering the long tortuous course of LCN dendrites and the high frequency of dendrodendritic contacts in the neuropil. Additional anatomical and physiological data are needed to further the understanding of the mechanisms of interaction of the TCPN and LCN in the cat motor thalamus.

Data concerning the TCPN-LCN relationships in the motor thalamus of species other than cat are even scarcer. In young rats both projection and local-circuit neurons in the VA were described in a Golgi impregnation study [11], but there are no published ultrastructural studies

---

Fig. 14. Low-power electron micrograph demonstrating a longitudinal section through a vesicle-containing dendrite (d) in the VA. Note the varicose outlines of the dendrite, dense packing of neurotubules in constricted parts, and accumulation of synaptic vesicles in varicose parts. Filled arrows point to SR boutons synapsing on varicose part; open arrow points to a dendrodendritic contact on a secondary TCPN dendrite. Note: here and in following figures demonstrating synaptic contacts arrows point from the postsynaptic side. Bar = 1 μm.

Fig. 15. Primary LCN dendrite (d) engaged in a synaptic contact with a secondary TCPN dendrite (D_2) in the VM. Note also an SR bouton that has an asymmetrical contact in the vicinity of the dendrodendritic synapse. Bar = 1 μm.

Fig. 16. High magnification of a dendrodendritic synapse. Note the symmetrical membrane specialization and presynaptic dense projections. Labeling as in Figure 15. Bar = 1 μm.

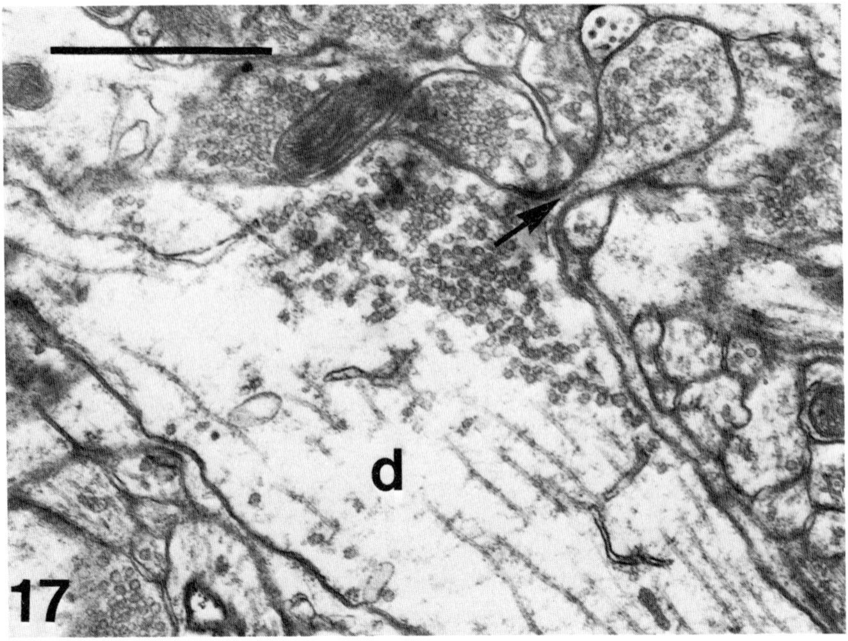

Fig. 17. Vesicle-containing dendrite (d) of LCN in the VL. Note a spine-like projection on a narrow neck (arrow) in continuity with d. Note also the accumulation of synaptic vesicles in both d and the spine-like projection. Bar = 1 μm.

on the motor thalamus of this species. Our unpublished observations in the rat motor nuclei did not reveal the presence of neurons with vesicle-containing dendrites. In light microscope immunocytochemical studies by Penny et al. [100] it was also noted that the rostral thalamic nuclei in several rodent species did not contain GAD-positive cells, whereas such cells were present in the geniculate nucleus of the same species. More recently, in an electrophysiological study, MacLeod and James [65] reported that they were not able to find electrophysiological evidence for the existence of the LCNs in the rat VM. It seems reasonable to assume, therefore, that GABAergic LCNs with vesicle-containing dendrites have not evolved in the motor thalamus of the rat and related rodent species.

To our knowledge there are no available Golgi impregnation studies in the motor thalamic nuclei of primates, although some data on their ultrastructure have been reported [3–6]. Harding and Powell [6], in their EM material from the ventrolateral thalamic region of the monkey, identified a population of small cells that gave rise to vesicle-containing dendrites. The latter were shown to participate in dendrodendritic synapses with TCPN dendrites as in the cat. Additionally, these dendrites were found to contact each other via unidirectional and reciprocal synapses. The latter finding implies that in the primate, unlike the cat, there is an anatomical substrate for direct communication between individual LCNs. Moreover, Harding and Powell [6] were able to identify an axon of one small cell and to show that it receives symmetrical synapses on its initial segment (see Fig. 3 in Harding and Powell [6]). Although no information on the origin of the latter contacts or on synaptic sites of LCN axons themselves is available, the above data suggest that one more level of LCN circuitry, different from that in nonprimate species, exists in the primate motor thalamus. The question of interest is whether the findings by Harding and Powell [6] represent the relationships characteristic for all motor thalamic nuclei in the primate. As seen in Figure 1, the subdivisions of the motor thalamus in primates are numerous and are distinct as regards their afferent-efferent connections. Even at the light microscope level in Nissl-stained preparations there are essential differences between the individual nuclei concerning the types and qualitative features of neurons present. The above authors stated that their EM specimens were mainly from two subdivisions, VLo and VLm, although they made generalizations in regard to the whole VL as well as the thalamus in general. It should be noted, however, that VLo is one of a few subdivisions where the population of small cells is numerous and is organized in a very specific pattern in relation to the larger cells. This cytoarchitectural feature makes the VLo nucleus easily distinguishable from surrounding subdivisions [45]. Therefore, until additional EM data on the monkey motor thalamus become available, a note of caution should be expressed about such generalizations.

5 SYNAPTOLOGY OF THE MOTOR THALAMUS

5.1 Types of Synaptic Boutons in the Normal Neuropil

There are only a few descriptive studies of the normal synaptic organization of the cat motor thalamus. Rinvik and Grofová [9] offered a classification of axon terminals found in the VA and VL based on several ultrastructural criteria, including shape and size of synaptic boutons and synaptic vesicles, and types of synaptic contacts formed by boutons. Five different types of boutons were recognized. Two of these contained round vesicles and formed asymmetrical contacts, but differed in size. One type was designated LR (*l*arge boutons with *r*ound synaptic vesicles) and another SR (*s*mall boutons with *r*ound synaptic vesicles). The SR terminals are the easiest to recognize in the normal neuropil owing to their small size and definitively asymmetrical contacts [Figs. 9, 15]. In LR boutons postsynaptic densities, although asymmetrical, are much less developed than in

SR boutons (Fig. 19). Also LR terminals, unlike SR type boutons, contain large numbers of mitochondria and form punta adherentes (Figs. 18, 19). Boutons of three other types (F1, F2, and F3) all contained pleomorphic vesicles and had symmetrical contacts, but they differed in other features including size. The F1 boutons were the largest, being 2.5 μm in average length, and they were also characterized by the presence of numerous mitochondria. F2 boutons were smaller and contained fewer mitochondria than F1 boutons. The third type, F3 boutons, were the smallest and had irregular outlines. The limitation of this otherwise excellent study [9] was that the authors did not differentiate between the VA and the VL, and therefore the differences in synaptic composition between the individual nuclei remained obscure.

In our study on the cat VM [101] both LR and SR boutons were also found in the normal neuropil (Figs. 9, 15), whereas the three F-type boutons could not be distinguished in this nucleus by the criteria described by Rinvik and Grofová [9] for VL and VA. Therefore, the synaptic boutons containing pleomorphic vesicles and forming symmetrical contacts were combined in one category designated the MP type (***m***edium-sized boutons with ***p***leomorphic vesicles) (Figs. 19, 20). All types of boutons with pleomorphic vesicles and symmetrical contacts in the cat VA, VM, and VL were shown to be GAD-positive (Figs. 33–35), which is strong evidence in favor of the inhibitory, GABAergic nature of these terminals [78].

In the neuropil of all three nuclei the SR-type boutons were the most numerous and formed synaptic contacts preferentially on the distal dendritic branches of TCPN as well as on LCN dendrites. Likewise the LR-type boutons contacted both cell types, but on TCPN dendrites they were found proximal to SR terminals. F1 terminals in the VA and VL were found only on the proximal dendritic shafts of TCPN [9], whereas MP-type terminals in the VM were seen to contact different-order dendritic branches of TCPN as well as some LCN dendrites [101].

The various types of axon terminals described in the cat motor thalamic nuclei may be found either to be establishing single contacts with postsynaptic structures or to be engaged in more complex synaptic relationships that involve several pre- and postsynaptic components. In all instances the postsynaptic components are represented by TCPN and LCN dendrites, and no axoaxonic synapses have been observed in any of the nuclei of the motor thalamus. The simplest arrangement is a serial synapse (Figs. 22, 25), where an axon terminal forms a contact on a GABAergic vesicle-containing dendrite of LCN, which in turn is presynaptic to a dendrite or in some instances the soma of TCPN [9,78]. In the cat only SR-type boutons are involved in these serial synapses (Fig. 26a).

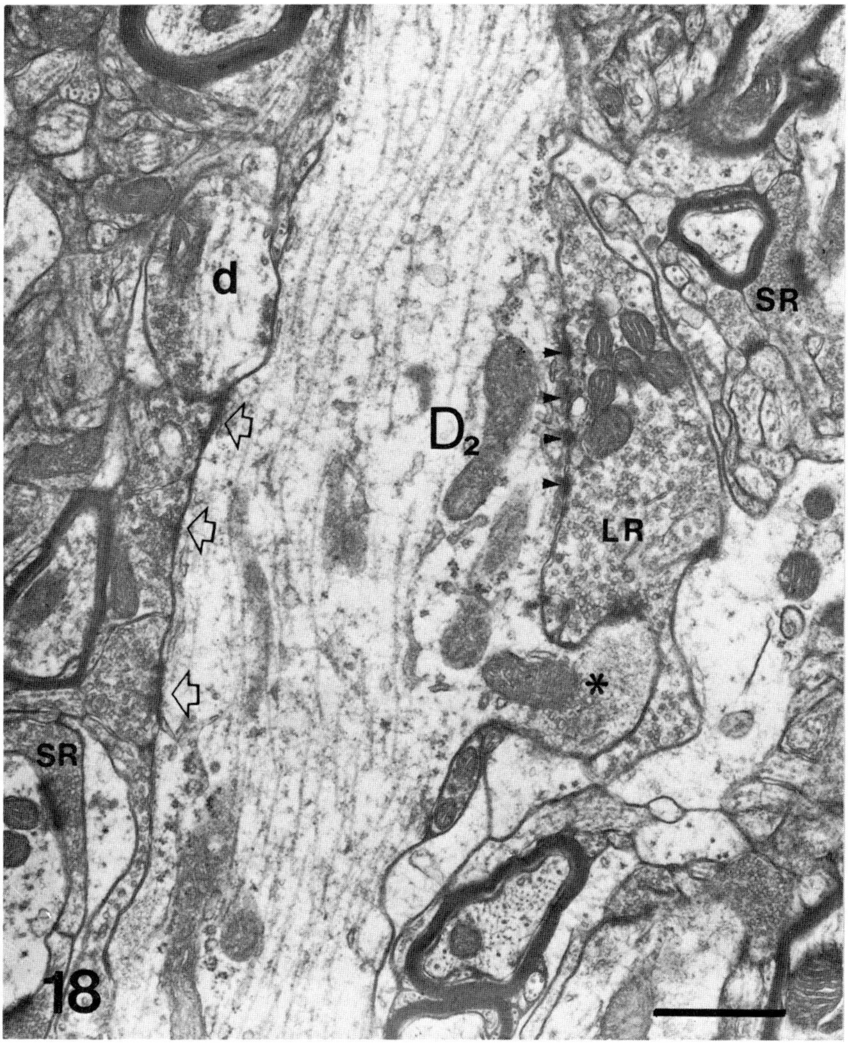

Fig. 18. Electron micrograph illustrating synaptic relationships of a secondary TCPN dendrite (D_2) in the extraglomerular neuropil of the VL. Asterisk marks a small projection from the surface of the dendrite. It contains a mitochondrion and dense filamentous substance and receives a synaptic contact from an LR bouton that is also attached to the main stem of the same dendrite by puncta adherentes (small arrowheads). On the opposite side of the dendrite is a row of three small boutons (probably F_3 type) containing small pleomorphic vesicles and forming symmetrical contacts (open arrows). Several SR boutons are also seen in surrounding neuropil. Bar = 1 μm.

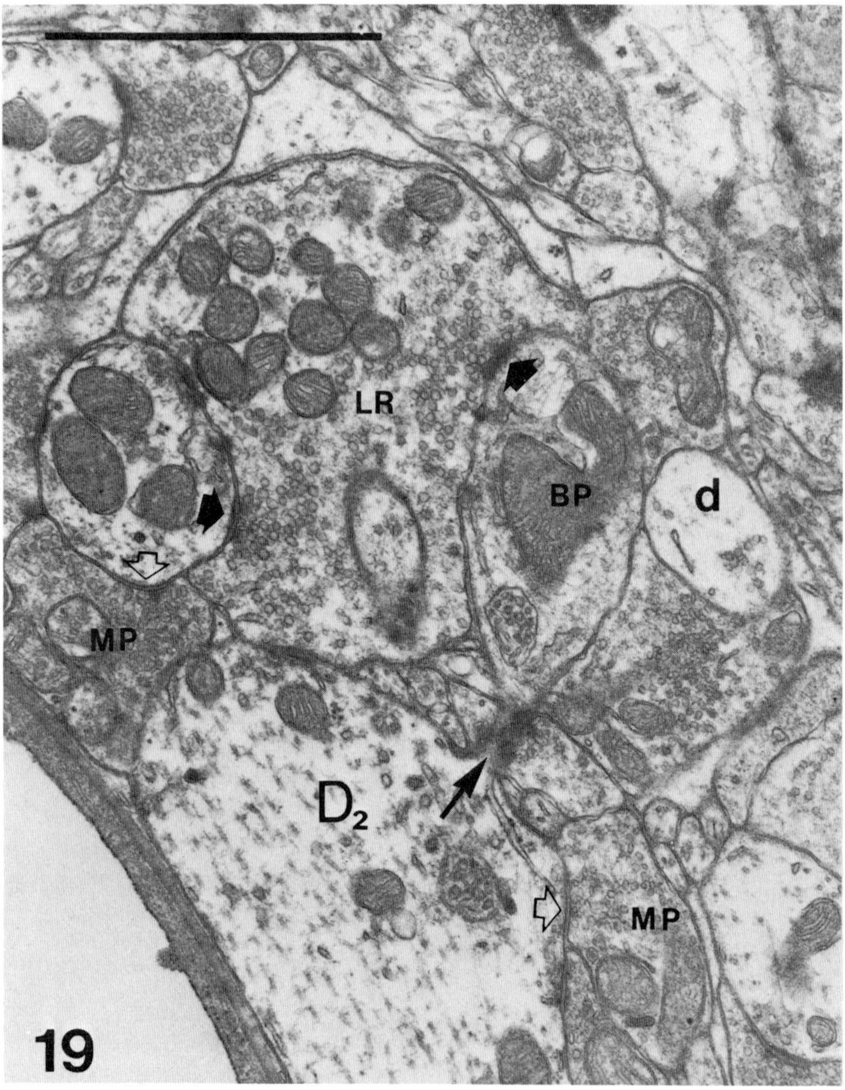

Fig. 19. Electron micrograph illustrating a part of a glomerulus associated with a secondary TCPN dendrite (D_2) and its bulbous protrusion (BP) in the VM. In the center is a large profile on an LR bouton that makes asymmetrical contacts (short black arrows) on BP and another small dendritic profile that is most likely a tertiary branch of the D_2. Seen as a part of the arrangement is a profile of an LCN dendrite (d) and two MP-type terminals forming symmetrical contacts (open arrows) on the TCPN dendrites. Long arrow points to connection between D_2 and BP. Bar = 1 μm.

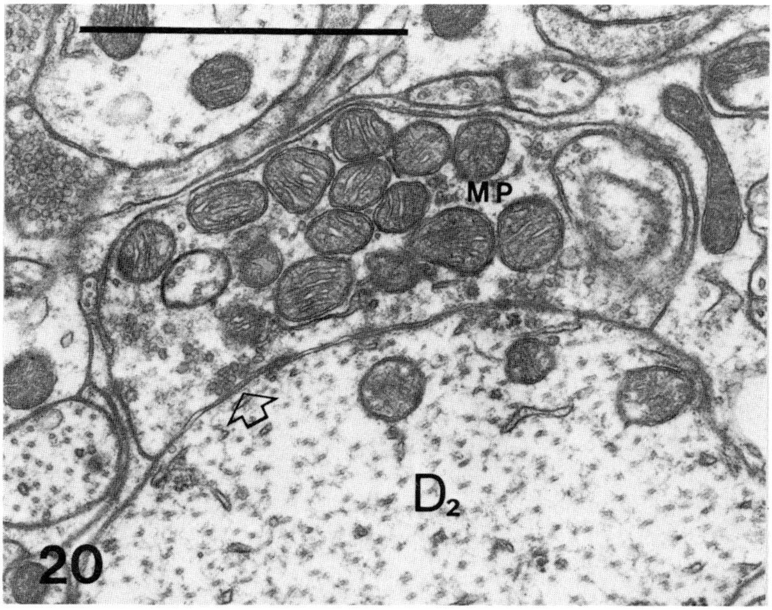

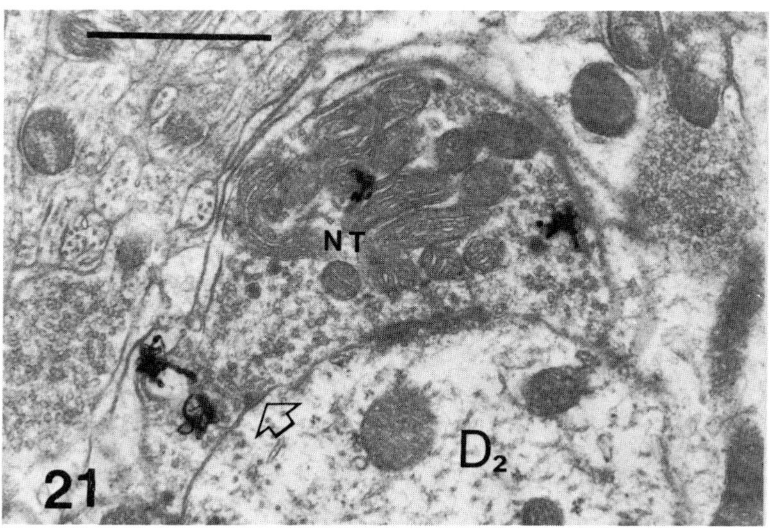

Fig. 20. Example of an MP-type terminal in the neuropil of the VM. The typical features of these boutons are pleomorphic synaptic vesicles and symmetrical contacts (open arrow). In most instances these profiles also display numerous mitochondria. D_2, secondary TCPN dendrite. Bar = 1 μm.

Fig. 21. Example of a nigral bouton (NT), similar to the MP-type terminal in Figure 20, that was labeled from a tritiated leucine injection in the substantia nigra. Other labeling as in Figure 20. Bar = 1 μm. Modified from Kultas-Ilinsky et al. [105].

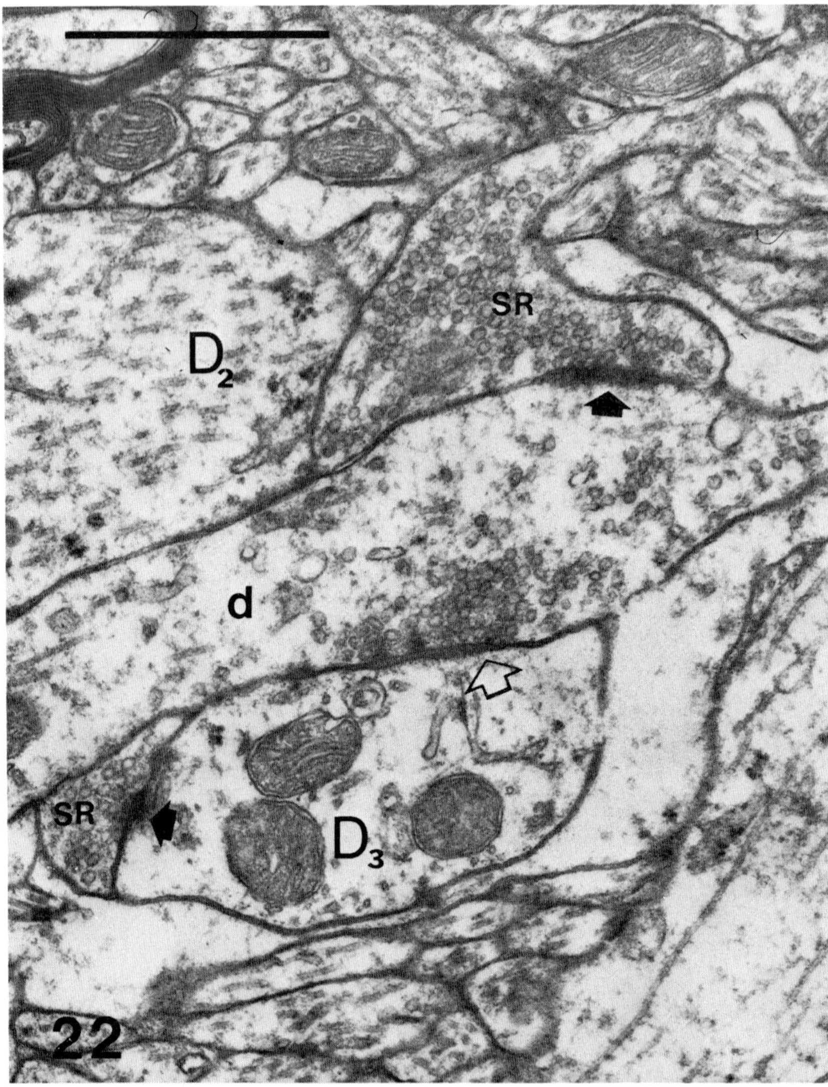

Fig. 22. Example of a serial synapse in the VA. The SR bouton in the center forms an asymmetrical synaptic contact (black arrow) on a vesicle-containing dendrite of LCN (d), which in turn synapses (open arrow) upon tertiary TCPN dendrite (D_3). The latter also receives a direct synapse from another SR bouton at the lower left (black arrow). D_2, secondary TCPN dendrite. Bar = 1 μm.

Another commonly found arrangement is a synaptic triad (Figs. 23, 24, 26b). In it an LR type bouton establishes synaptic contacts on both TCPN and LCN dendrites, the latter in turn forming a symmetrical contact on the same TCPN dendrite [9,78,99]. The most complex type of synaptic arrangement is a glomerulus. Glomeruli in the motor thalamus are usually formed by a group of synaptic boutons arranged around a secondary or higher-order dendritic branch of TCPN, its bulbous protrusion, and numerous profiles of vesicle-containing dendrites (Fig. 27). Several LR-type boutons are commonly found in a single glomerulus, each of them forming a triad with LCN and TCPN dendrites. It was observed that MP-type terminals in the VM [101], and F2 and F3 terminals in the VA and VL [9] also participate in these complexes. The glomeruli are surrounded by several layers of astroglial processes that isolate them from the surrounding extraglomerular neuropil.

It should be mentioned that the glomeruli do not represent a unique feature of the motor nuclei, since these complex synaptic assemblies have been described in almost all nuclei of the cat thalamus [8,91,102–104]. Within the motor thalamus, however, differences in the number and composition of glomeruli have been noted between individual subdivisions. For example, in the neuropil of the VL, glomeruli are very frequent, whereas in the VM and VA they are relatively rare [78]. Furthermore, glomeruli in VL contain more LR profiles than those in the VA and VM. On the other hand, the glomeruli in the latter two nuclei contain medium to large GAD-positive boutons of basal ganglia origin [105], whereas in the VL the most conspicuous GAD-positive component of glomeruli is represented by numerous profiles of LCN dendrites [78].

No published data are available on the ultrastructure of the rat motor nuclei. Our unpublished observations indicate that the basic types of synaptic boutons described for the cat such as SR, LR, and MP are also found in the rat motor nuclei (Figs. 28, 29). However, owing to the absence of LCNs with vesicle-containing dendrites, none of the complex synaptic arrangements described above are present in the rat motor thalamus.

In the monkey, the data on the normal ultrastructure of the ventral lateral region of the thalamus come almost exclusively from the studies by Harding [3–5] and Harding and Powell [6]. The types of synaptic boutons recognized by these authors were basically the same as those described in the cat by Rinvik and Grofová [9]. The SR and LR boutons generally had the same ultrastructural features and comparable termination sites; F-type boutons with pleomorphic vesicles and symmetrical contacts were also present. All types of axon terminals were found to participate in complex synaptic arrangements, such as serial synapses, triads, and glomeruli. The unique feature of the primate motor thalamus appears to be the high

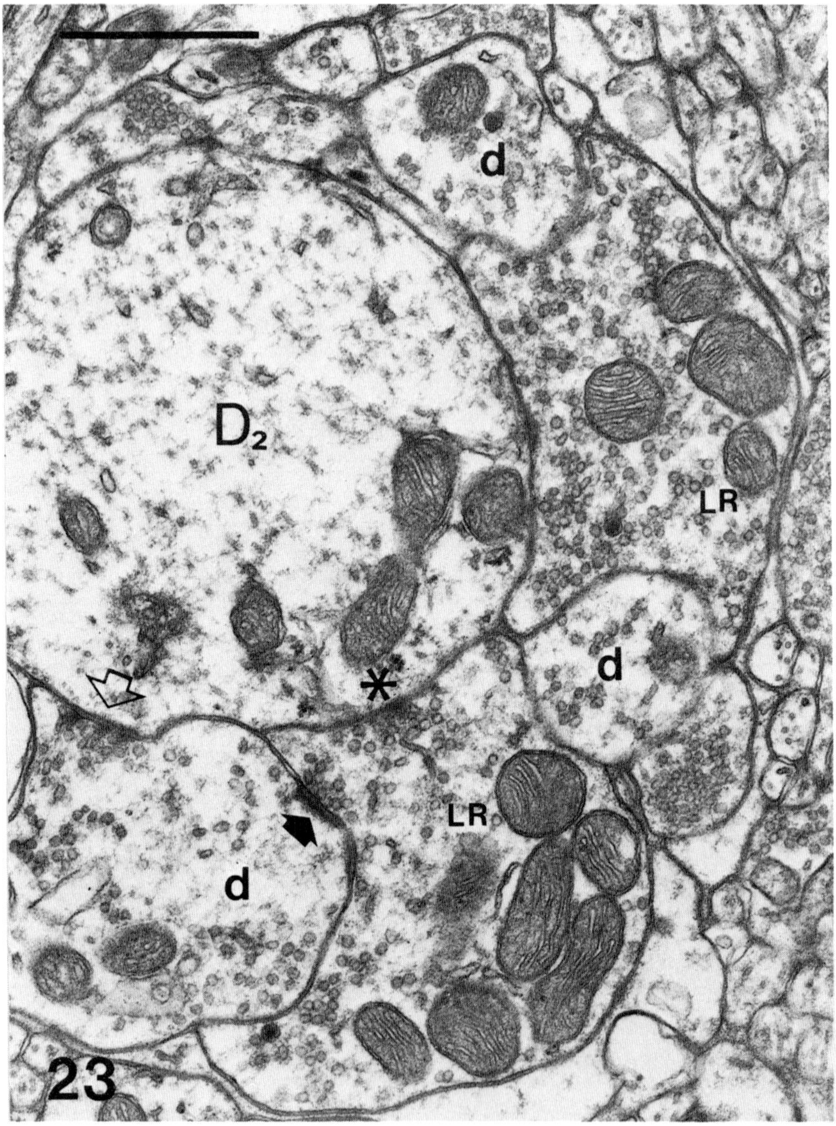

Fig. 23. Two LR profiles apposing a secondary TCPN dendrite (D_2) and several vesicle-containing profiles of LCN dendrites (d) in the VA. The lower LR bouton is engaged in a triad. Its contact with D_2 sectioned tangentially is indicated by an asterisk, the contact with d is shown by black arrow, and the contact between d and D_2 is indicated by an open arrow. Bar = 1 μm.

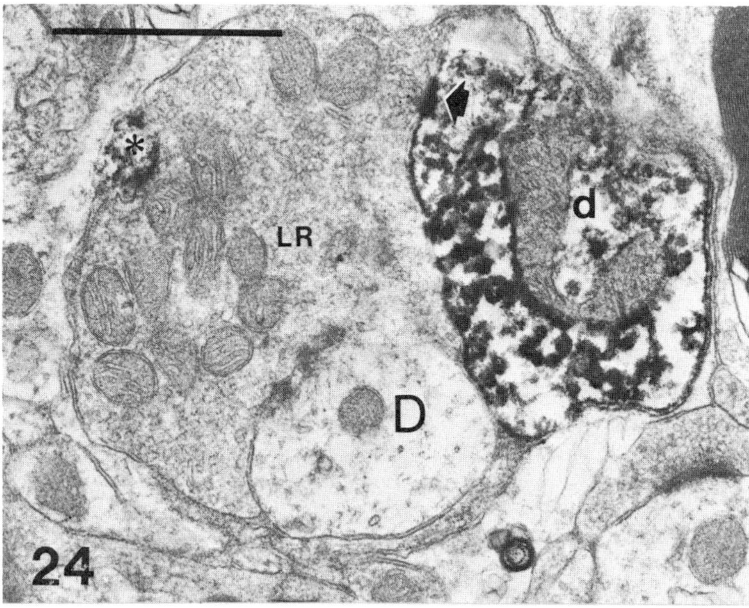

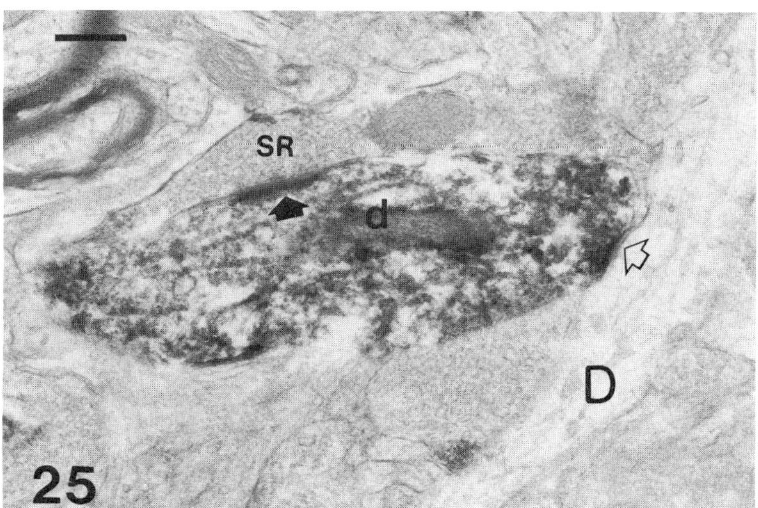

Figs. 24, 25. Examples of GAD-immunoreactive dendrites in the neuropil of the VA. Modified from Kultas-Ilinsky et al. [78].

Fig. 24. An LR bouton is associated with two GAD-positive profiles that belong to LCN dendrites (d and asterisk), and a TCPN dendrite (D). The arrow points to synaptic contact between the LR bouton and d. This relationship is most likely part of a triad as in Figure 23. Bar = 1 μm.

Fig. 25. A serial synapse between an SR bouton, a GAD-positive, vesicle-containing LCN dendrite (d), and a TCPN dendrite (D). Black arrow points to asymmetrical contact between SR and d; open arrow points to symmetrical contact between d and D. The relationship is similar to that demonstrated in Figure 22. Bar = 1 μm.

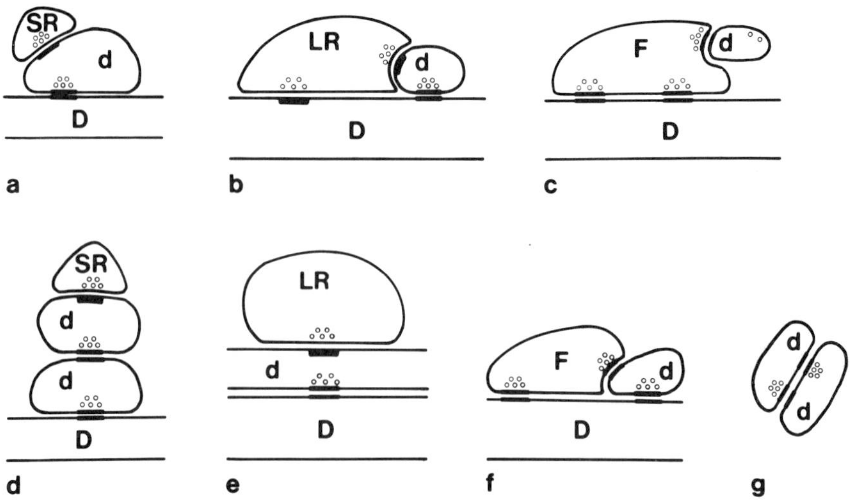

Fig. 26. Diagram illustrating various types of complex synaptic arrangements in the cat (a–c) and monkey (a–g) motor thalamus. Data for monkey are compiled from Harding and Powell [6]. a, Serial synapse with SR type bouton; b, a triad with LR bouton; c, F or MP terminal contacting both TCPN and LCN dendrites; d, sequential serial synapse with SR bouton; e, serial synapse with LR bouton; f, triad with F bouton; g, reciprocal synapse between two LCN dendrites. D, Dendrites of thalamocortical projection neurons (TCPN); d, dendrites of local-circuit neurons (LCN). The asymmetrical synaptic contacts are indicated by thicker lines on postsynaptic side. The symmetrical contacts are indicated by two parallel lines of equal thickness.

degree of complexity of these synaptic arrays. For example, in addition to simple serial synapses (Fig. 26a, e), a more complex variant called a sequential serial synapse was observed. In the latter, several sequential dendrodendritic synapses formed by LCN dendrites were imposed between the SR or LR bouton and a TCPN dendrite (Fig. 26d). The glomeruli in the primate also seem to have a more complex organization: they contain a higher number of LCN dendrites and triads formed by LR boutons; additionally, sequential serial synapses and reciprocal synapses (Fig. 26g) participate in these complexes. Finally, a different type of a triad, where an axon terminal is represented by an F-type bouton and all three synaptic contacts are symmetrical, has also been described in the glomerular and extraglomerular neuropil in the monkey motor thalamus (Fig. 26f). Note that in the cat similar F-type boutons are found in diads only (Fig. 26c).

Although data on the normal ultrastructural organization of the neuropil of the motor thalamus are far from complete, those that are available point to a general trend—namely, that the degree of complexity

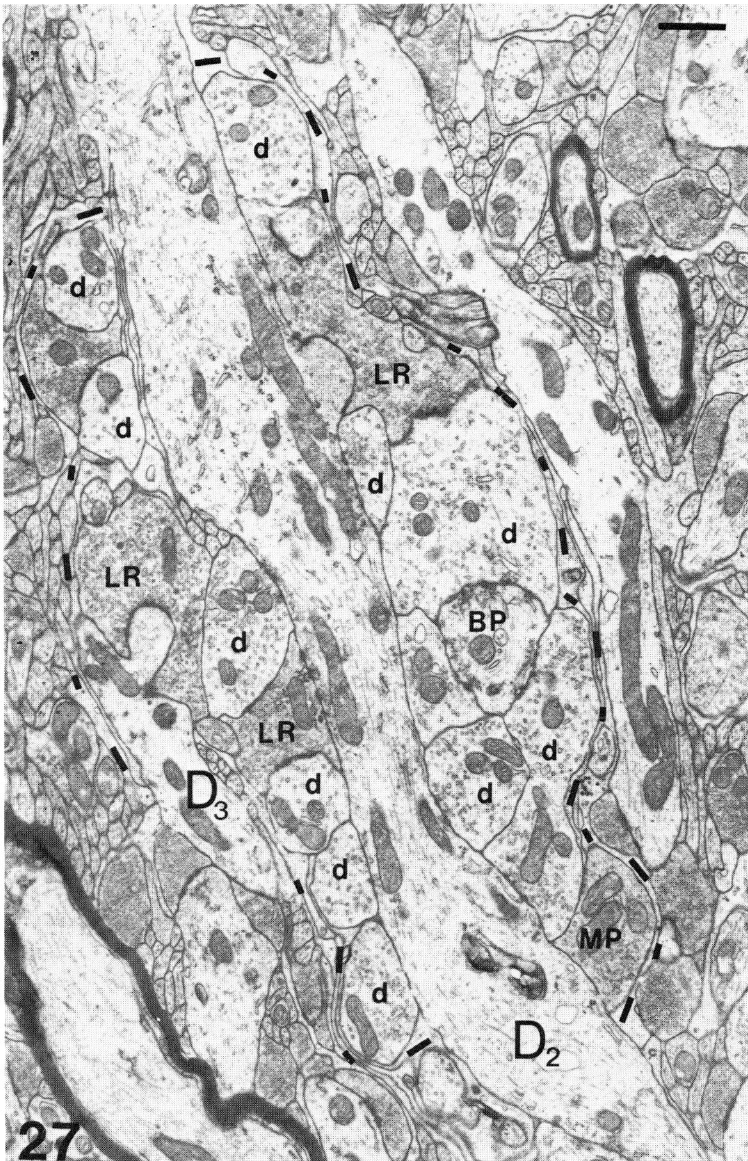

Fig. 27. An example of a longitudinally sectioned glomerulus in the lateral posterior VM formed by secondary (D_2) and tertiary (D_3) dendritic branches of TCPN, the bulbous process of D_2 (BP), and numerous profiles of vesicle-containing dendrites (d). Note the presence of several LR boutons and one MP bouton. The incomplete glial sheath around the glomerulus is indicated by a dashed line. Bar = 1 μm.

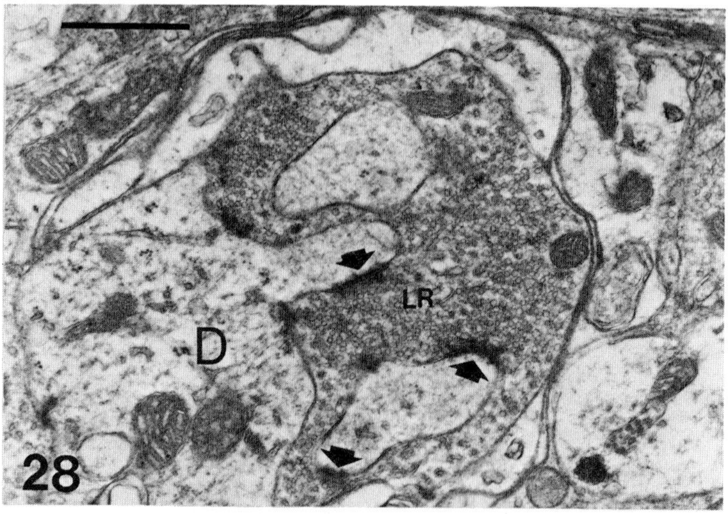

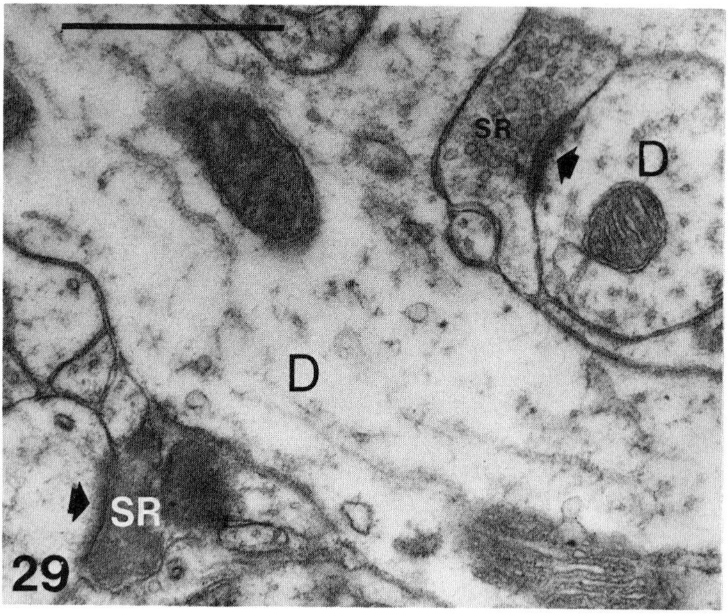

Figs. 28, 29. Examples of axon terminals in the rat motor thalamus.

Fig. 28. An LR-type bouton associated with a dendrite and its three spine-like processes, two of which receive asymmetrical synapses (arrows). Bar = 1 μm.

Fig. 29. A normal SR bouton forming an asymmetrical synapse on a small-diameter dendrite (D) at upper right, and a similar SR profile at lower left degenerating after ablation of the motor cortex. Arrows point to asymmetrical contacts. Bar = 1 μm. From Kultas-Ilinsky et al. [119].

of synaptic organization increases with evolutionary specialization and LCN dendrites are instrumental in this. It is striking how little difference there is between the basic types of synaptic boutons found in the three species but also how complex synaptic arrangements become in phylogenetically advanced species. The complexity of the synaptic arrangements seems to be directly proportional to the number of variants of synaptic relationships that engage LCN dendrites.

Although intracellular studies on the mechanisms by which these complex synaptic arrangements operate are lacking, a number of possibilities have been put forward for both motor and other thalamic nuclei where similar relationships exist. For instance, Purpura [106] has proposed that dendrodendritic synapses between the LCN and TCPN may be responsible for the inhibitory postsynaptic potentials (IPSPs) that usually follow the short initial excitatory postsynaptic potential (EPSP) recorded from TCPN after stimulation of primary afferents. This suggestion was based on observations that the time interval between the initial EPSP and following IPSPs was too short for other, longer circuits to become involved in the response. It has also been suggested [107] that, owing to the remoteness of the majority of dendrodendritic synapses from somata of the parent cells, they may operate as separate units independent of the activities of the other dendrites or even of somata of the TCPN. Since the majority of dendrodendritic synapses are usually associated with axodendritic synapses formed by different type boutons, they are ideally situated to modify the activity that is transmitted from these axon terminals to projection neurons. For example, triadic synapses may modify the tonic activity arriving via LR-type afferent terminals into a phasic activity that is received by projection neuron dendrites [108,109]. Thus, one can further speculate that the functional significance of the evolutionary trend mentioned above is to provide a finer regulation of the afferent input to thalamocortical neurons, which in turn should result in finer tuning of their output activity.

5.2 Identification of the Afferent Origin of Axon Terminals in the Motor Thalamus

5.2.1 Methodological considerations. A number of experimental approaches have been used to determine the afferent origin of axon terminals observed in the normal neuropil. The techniques employed utilize anterograde degeneration or anterograde transport of markers such as HRP or tritiated amino acids. Each of these techniques has a number of advantages and drawbacks. The latter, when not taken into account, may easily lead to significant misinterpretations. Therefore a few comments on some technical aspects are called for at the beginning of this section.

The simplest and fastest way of marking the terminals of an afferent system is by causing their degeneration following lesioning of the appropriate structure, and then identifying the boutons by the degeneration features displayed. Different degenerative features of synaptic boutons have been observed in various brain regions (see Kultas-Ilinsky et al. [99] for references). The most frequently described is the "dark" or "electron-dense" type of degeneration, during which there is a swelling of synaptic vesicles, darkening of axoplasmic matrix, and considerable shrinkage of the terminal. Another pattern of degeneration is the "filamentous" type; it is characterized by the disappearance of synaptic vesicles and the presence of large numbers of microfilaments that fill the whole terminal. The third degeneration pattern is the "electron-lucent" or "pale" type, and is characterized by clumping, swelling, and finally disappearance of synaptic vesicles and all other axoplasmic organelles, accompanied by enormous swelling of the terminal itself. The causes of these different degeneration patterns remain obscure. In earlier literature there was a tendency to believe that a certain degeneration pattern is specific for each particular afferent system and therefore can be used as an additional means of identification of the pathway. However, it has already been noted (see Section 5.2.4 and Figs. 30, 31) that the same pathway can display more than one degeneration pattern, and so the value of the latter as an identification criterion is questionable.

In general the disadvantages inherent in the use of the degeneration technique are that 1) degeneration significantly alters the ultrastructural features of the terminals (i.e., size and shape of synaptic boutons and synaptic vesicles), so that the identification of degenerating boutons with their counterparts in normal tissue is not always unequivocal; 2) quantitative studies, especially those related to the density of particular types of terminals in the tissue, are hindered since not all terminals of the same pathway degenerate simultaneously; only a portion of the total population of boutons identified by degenerative features can be observed in the tissue at each given postlesion survival time [110]; 3) if electrolytic lesions are used, the population of degenerating boutons of the afferent pathway under consideration may be contaminated by the presence of terminals of another unrelated pathway whose fibers happen to pass through or close to the lesioned structure. The latter consideration is especially important, and ignoring it may lead to significant misinterpretations (see Section 5.2.4). However, at present this drawback can be overcome by the use of chemical lesioning agents, such as neurotoxic amino acids (i.e., ibotenic or kainic), which in appropriate concentrations cause only degeneration of neuronal somata, leaving fibers of passage intact [111–117]. Ibotenic acid may be especially useful in studying the relationships of closely situated small nuclei since, unlike kainic acid, its diffusion is very limited and can be easily controlled. However, not many ultrastructural studies with this lesioning agent are available.

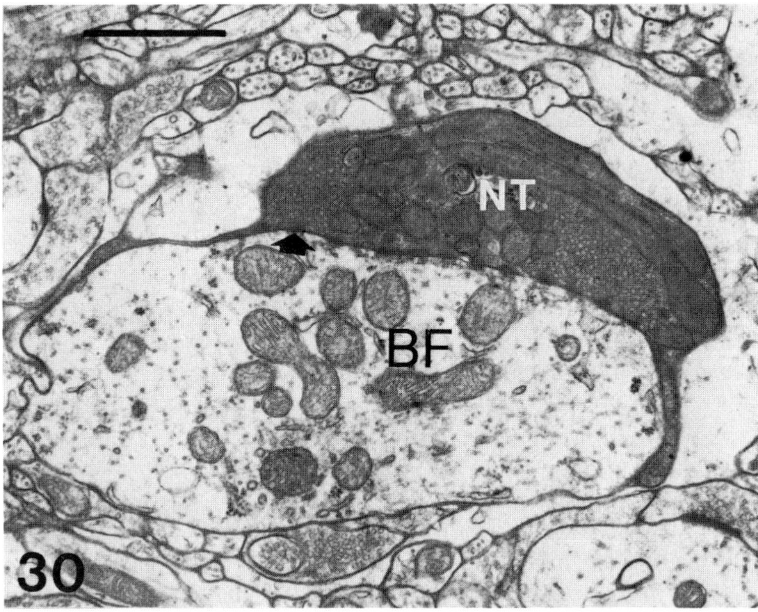

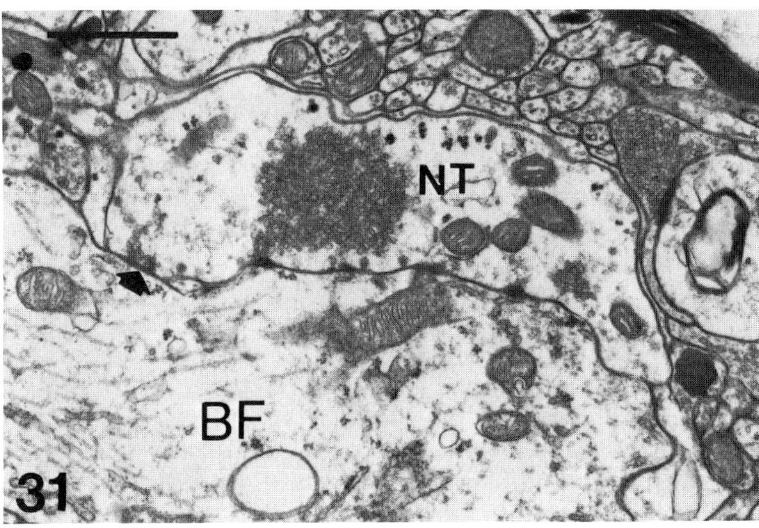

Figs. 30, 31. Examples of degeneration features of axon terminals in the cat VM after injections of ibotenic acid in substantia nigra pars reticularis.

Fig. 30. Electron-dense degeneration of a nigral terminal (NT) that synapses (arrow) at a cross-sectioned bifurcation (BF) of a primary TCPN dendrite. Bar = 1 μm.

Fig. 31. Electron-lucent degeneration displayed by a nigral terminal (NT) synapsing (arrow) at an obliquely sectioned bifurcation site of a primary dendrite (BF). Both nigral boutons are from the same experiment (6 days postlesion survival) and from the same thin section. Bar = 1 μm.

The limitations of using HRP as a tracer in light microscope studies have been mentioned earlier (see Section 3.4) and the criticism expressed concerning its uptake by lesioned fibers is equally applicable to ultrastructural studies. Additionally, two other pitfalls should be considered: one is that the histochemical procedure for HRP is less sensitive in the higher pH range which is favorable for tissue preservation [118]; the other stems from the often observed phenomenon that the dense reaction product may obscure the ultrastructural features of a labeled structure. Thus, with the EM-HRP techniques available at present, the two goals of achieving maximal labeling of the pathway and maintaining an acceptable degree of preservation and resolution of the ultrastructure are in conflict.

The most reliable technique for labeling afferent terminals is EM autoradiography of anterogradely transported amino acids. The advantages are many and include specificity, an excellent preservation of normal ultrastructure, and the possibility of performing quantitative studies. The main drawback of the technique is that it is labor-intensive and time-consuming, since exposure times may last for up to 6 months.

We have found that the use of a combination of the techniques on a system of interest is the most beneficial approach, since the pitfalls of individual methodologies balance out and the information obtained is more complete. The terminals of several afferent systems that have been ultrastructurally identified in the motor thalamus by means of the techniques discussed are described below.

5.2.2 Corticothalamic afferents. The degeneration technique was used for identification of terminals of corticothalamic afferents in the cat VA and VL by Grofová and Rinvik [2], in the monkey ventrolateral thalamus by Harding and Powell [6], and in the rat motor thalamus by Kultas-Ilinsky et al. [119]. In all species it was found that the SR-type boutons degenerated after cortical lesions and in all instances they displayed features of dark degeneration (Fig. 29). Degenerating SR boutons were usually found in clusters and degeneration of both myelinated and unmyelinated axons was also observed as a result of cortical lesions. These features of cortical afferent terminals seem to be similar in all thalamic nuclei where the cortical input has been studied [120]. The consistency of these findings in different nuclei as well as different species allows one to ascribe with reasonable confidence a cortical origin to all SR boutons found in neuropil and thus analyze the distribution of cortical afferents on different types of neurons.

When all available data on these terminals are put together, it is apparent that the cortical input is directed primarily to the distal dendritic branches of TCPN, where these terminals dominate. In the cat motor nuclei the cortical boutons are not found on primary dendrites or somata of TCPN, and on secondary dendritic branches they are infrequent. The

LCNs in all three motor nuclei also receive substantial cortical input. The cortical terminals are found either singly on LCN dendrites or form a constituent part of serial synapses in the cat and sequential serial synapses in the monkey. In the cat VL these boutons have also been observed in contact with LCN somata [78].

These findings indicate that TCPN receive two kinds of input from the cortex, one direct and the other indirect, i.e. mediated by LCN dendrites. The asymmetrical contacts displayed by these terminals are in accordance with the excitatory nature of the corticothalamic afferents demonstrated in electrophysiological studies [70,121–123]. The input mediated by LCN dendrites should be inhibitory because of the GABAergic nature of LCNs. Such an inhibitory cortical influence would be distributed to TCPN dendrites as well as their somata via dendrodendritic or dendrosomatic serial synapses engaging SR-type boutons. Indeed IPSPs have also been recorded after electrical stimulation of cortical afferents [122,123]. The most common effect of the activation of corticothalamic pathways is the bursting rhythmic discharges of TCPN described by several investigators (see Steriade and Deschênes [73] for references). In recent studies with intracellular recordings in the cat motor thalamus, it was shown that this response of TCPN consists of several components, each of which is associated with different ion currents and occurs at different levels of the somadendritic membrane of TCPN [73,124]. It was suggested that cells of the reticular thalamic nucleus, as well as local-circuit neurons, may participate in different components of this response. However, as stated earlier (Section 3.4) there is no solid evidence in favor of reticular nucleus projections to the motor thalamus. Nevertheless, it seems that the known synaptic relationships of cortical afferents with TCPN and LCN dendrites by themselves provide an adequate anatomical substrate for these physiological phenomena. Thus, the initial component of the corticothalamic response, described as short-latency EPSP of remote dendritic origin by Steriade and Deschênes [73], can be mediated by direct synapses formed by cortical terminals on tertiary dendrites of TCPN. The second component, determined as Cl^--dependent IPSP in the perisomatic region, can be the result of activation of serial synapses composed by SR boutons → GABAergic LCN dendrites → TCPN soma. The third component of the response, which is a long-lasting hyperpolarization mediated by CA^{2+}-dependent K^+ currents and is ascribed to more proximal dendrites, may involve serial synapses formed by SR boutons → GABAergic LCN dendrites → secondary TCPN dendrites. It should be noted that synapses of cortical afferents on the somata and proximal dendrites of LCNs described in the VL [78] may also contribute to this component of corticothalamic response. These would cause the excitation of LCNs, which in turn could prolong the inhibition of TCPN.

There are certain aspects of the organization of corticothalamic afferents that are still unclear. One of these is especially relevant in the nuclei with multiple cortical targets, such as VA and VM. It is not known whether corticothalamic projections from the different cortical areas converge on the same cells in these thalamic nuclei or whether projections from each cortical area are targeted exclusively to those neuronal populations that give rise to the respective thalamocortical projections.

Another aspect about which little is known is the neurotransmitter that is utilized by the corticothalamic afferents to the motor nuclei. Evidence has been accumulating, however, to suggest a role for glutamate as neurotransmitter in corticofugal pathways, including corticothalamic [125–127].

5.2.3 Cerebellothalamic afferents. In the cat, cerebellar terminals have been identified in the motor thalamus by both degeneration and EM autoradiography techniques [10,99,128]. All studies agree that the cerebellar terminals are of LR type, since both degenerating and labeled boutons are usually of large size with a high content of synaptic vesicles and mitochondria and form asymmetrical contacts. In the lesioning experiments they have been shown to display either filamentous [10] or all three types of degeneration [99]. Differences in the distribution and synaptic sites of cerebellar boutons in individual motor nuclei have been observed [99]. For example, cerebellar terminals identified in the VM after electrolytic lesions in the brachium conjunctivum were found to synapse on the LCN dendrites as frequently as, if not more often than, on TCPN dendrites. This indicates that cerebellar input in the VM is distributed more or less equally between the two types of neurons. In the same study in the VM it was demonstrated that cerebellar terminals do not synapse on primary TCPN dendrites but are found mainly on secondary and tertiary branches and are sometimes located at the bifurcation sites of the latter. Moreover, cerebellar boutons were frequently observed in triads, both in glomeruli and in extraglomerular neuropil. These results were very similar to observations on degenerating cerebellar boutons in the cat VA and VL [10]. Another study [128] using EM autoradiographic identification of cerebellar projections originating from two individual cerebellar nuclei, dentate and fastigial, confirmed synaptic sites of cerebellar boutons in the VA and VM. It was also shown that in the medial VL the termination sites of dentate efferents were somewhat different, in that they were frequently found on primary dendrites of TCPN. The main drawback of this quantitative study was that it was done on a relatively small sample of boutons labeled only from dentate and fastigial nuclei and on limited regions of the motor thalamus. There are no similar data available on the terminals of afferents from nucleus interpositus.

In the above-mentioned EM autoradiography study [128] a quantitative analysis of the ultrastructural features of the axon terminals from two cerebellar nuclei was also performed. It was found that boutons of dentate and fastigial origin can be differentiated by the size and shape of their synaptic vesicles in spite of the fact that they belong to one general class of LR boutons. This demonstrated that quantitative analysis of ultrastructural features of synaptic boutons can bring out subtle morphological differences that are not apparent qualitatively; it also pointed to the existence in the motor thalamus of several subpopulations of LR boutons. The terminals of projections from nucleus interpositus, when similarly studied, may reveal their own unique fine-structural features, as well as synaptic sites different from those of dentate and fastigial terminals. Moreover, terminals of some other possible afferent inputs (see Section 3.4) that have not as yet been ultrastructurally identified may also belong to the same broad category of LR boutons. This is likely, since LR-type boutons are not a unique feature of the motor thalamus. Similar characteristics have been attributed to terminals of primary afferents in other thalamic nuclei of various species, including lemniscal fibers in the somatosensory nuclear complex and retinal fibers in the lateral geniculate nucleus (see Harding and Powell [6] for references).

In regard to the monkey motor thalamus, terminals degenerating following cerebellar lesions have also been shown to be of the LR type [6]. In the region of the motor thalamus studied, the cerebellar boutons were found mainly in glomeruli, where they were engaged in complex synaptic arrangements such as triads and sequential serial synapses. These data are the only ones available on the ultrastructure of cerebellar boutons in the primate. However, they may not reflect in full the synaptic organization of the cerebellar input in the monkey. According to Harding and Powell [6], their samples were taken mainly from the VLm and VLo, and therefore the subdivisions that are the major recipients of cerebellar input, such as VPLo, area X, VLc (see Fig. 1, and Section 3.1), were not analyzed. Thus their observations on the cerebellar terminals are limited to VLm since, according to light microscope data, VLo does not receive cerebellar input (see Section 3.1). Further quantitative studies on the organization of the cerebellar input to the motor thalamus of the monkey are needed, therefore, to appreciate the organization of this afferent input in individual nuclear subdivisions.

As in the case of SR boutons, asymmetrical contacts of LR boutons of cerebellar origin correlate well with the excitatory nature of this input [63–65,70–72,129,130]. With intracellular recordings, monosynaptic short-latency EPSPs or EPSP-IPSP sequences are usually recorded from TCPNs after stimulation of cerebellar nuclei or the brachium conjuctivum [70].

Polysynaptic long-latency excitation and long-latency inhibiton were also observed [129,131]. Such a variable response may result from the fact that cerebellar input is received by both TCPN and LCN, and it also may reflect the different types of synaptic relationships in which cerebellar terminals are engaged (i.e., single terminals, triads in extraglomerular neuropil, and complex relationships within the glomeruli).

In the latter two arrangements the GABAergic LCNs play an essential role. However, no axoaxonic contacts with participation of LR boutons or any other axon terminals have been found in the motor thalamus. In this context the recently postulated mechanism of action of the cerebellar input engaging axoaxonic contacts is not supported by anatomical data [132].

Several aspects of the organization of the cerebellar input to the motor thalamus require further exploration. One is the lack of ultrastructural data on terminals of projections from nucleus interpositus. Another concerns the relationships between afferents from individual nuclei of the cerebellum. Anatomical data concerning the convergence of inputs from different cerebellar nuclei on the same cells of the motor thalamus are virtually nonexistent. Electrophysiological studies have demonstrated that convergence of the cerebellar input from all three nuclei, or different combinations of them, occurs on the individual neurons of the VL [131]. Differences in the topographical distribution of cells receiving certain combinations of converging cerebellar inputs was noted along with the diversity of electrophysiological effects elicited on the same cells from stimulation of various combinations of cerebellar nuclei [131].

On the basis of data discussed in this section, it may be postulated that future anatomical studies will show that fibers from individual cerebellar nuclei have different modes of termination even when converging on the same thalamic cells, and that the role of LCNs in mediating the input from individual cerebellar nuclei to different subdivisions of the motor thalamus differs substantially. Finally, very limited data are available concerning the neurotransmitter(s) mediating the cerebellar input to the thalamus. Some earlier studies based on indirect evidence suggested acetylcholine (ACh) as a putative neurotransmitter in this system [133]. In a recent study in the rat VM, where this hypothesis was tested, the results were equivocal and suggested a dual role for ACh both as a transmitter and a modulator [134]. Moreover, some indirect evidence has been reported recently suggesting that glutamate may be a neurotransmitter in some cerebellothalamic fibers [132].

5.2.4 Basal ganglia afferents (pallidal and nigral). *Pallidal afferents* have been identified in the cat thalamus by both degeneration [2] and EM autoradiography techniques [28,105]. Grofová and Rinvik [2] were the first to present a detailed description of the ultrastructural features and synaptic sites of pallidal boutons in the cat VA and VL. They found that after lesions in the entopeduncular nucleus F1-type boutons displayed an electron-lucent degeneration. The pallidal axons, after loosing their myelin sheath, formed several "en passant" synapses, mainly on proximal dendrites of TCPN. Recently, their findings have been confirmed and further expanded in a quantitative EM autoradiography study [105]. The latter findings demonstrated that in the VA and VM, in addition to synaptic contacts on somata and primary and secondary TCPN dendrites, pallidal terminals also form a limited number of contacts on tertiary TCPN dendrites and on LCN dendrites. The ultrastructural features of pallidal boutons were fairly consistent. Although they varied in size from medium to large, in most instances they displayed large numbers of mitochondria and puncta adherentes. They contained pleomorphic vesicles and formed exclusively symmetrical contacts (Fig. 32). The latter is in agreement with electrophysiological findings that demonstrate the inhibitory nature of this input [68,69].

Two publications are available that describe degeneration of pallidal terminals in the motor thalamus of primates [6,135]. Nitecka et al. [135] studied pallidal afferents in the VA and VLo of the squirrel monkey. They found that a variety of types of synaptic boutons degenerated after electrolytic lesions in the globus pallidus. These degenerating boutons were designated as types ILR, IIEF, IVMR, and 5SO. The ILR type was described as boutons with asymmetrical contacts and pleomorphic vesicles, whereas type IIEF was considered a counterpart of the F1-type of Rinvik and Grofová [2,9]. Analysis of the electron micrographs presented by Nitecka et al. [135] reveals that the ultrastructural features of the boutons in the two categories (ILR and IIEF) are remarkably similar. Both are of relatively large size, contain pleomorphic vesicles, form symmetrical contacts, and display large numbers of mitochondria and puncta adherentes. In other words, the terminals degenerating after pallidal lesions in the monkey (*Saimiri sciureus*) are almost identical to the boutons identified as terminals of pallidal origin in the cat [2,105]. The reason why the investigators discriminated an additional category of these boutons (ILR) must have been that the numerous puncta adherentes typical of these terminals were interpreted as asymmetric contacts (see Fig. 2 in Nitecka et al. [135]). On the other hand, both IVMR and 5SO terminals degenerating after pallidal lesions [135] had features typical of SR boutons (i.e., characteristic of cortical afferent terminals). The degeneration of these boutons was most likely due to involvement in the lesion of corticothalamic fibers passing through the internal capsule in the vicinity of the globus pallidus.

In another study on the monkey (*Macaca mulatta*) motor thalamus by Harding and Powell [6], the boutons degenerating after pallidal lesions were described as belonging solely to the SR type, and according to their

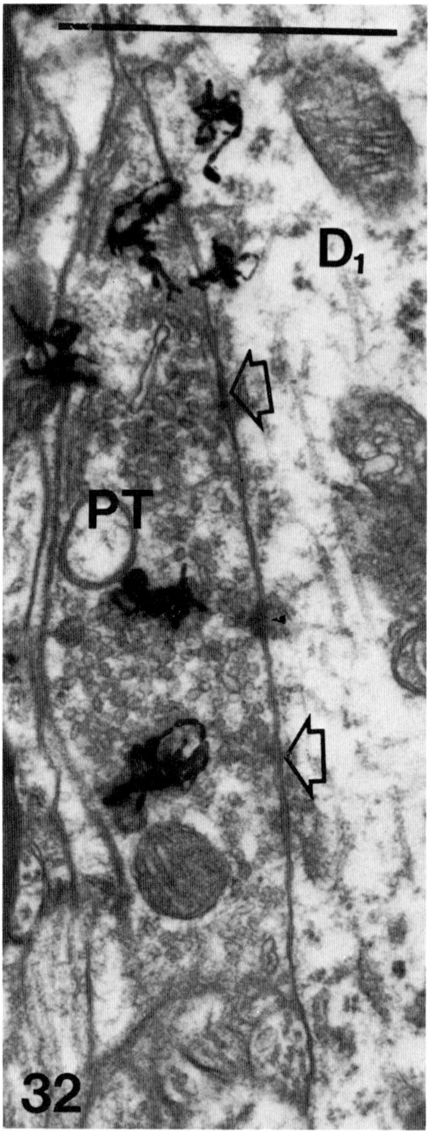

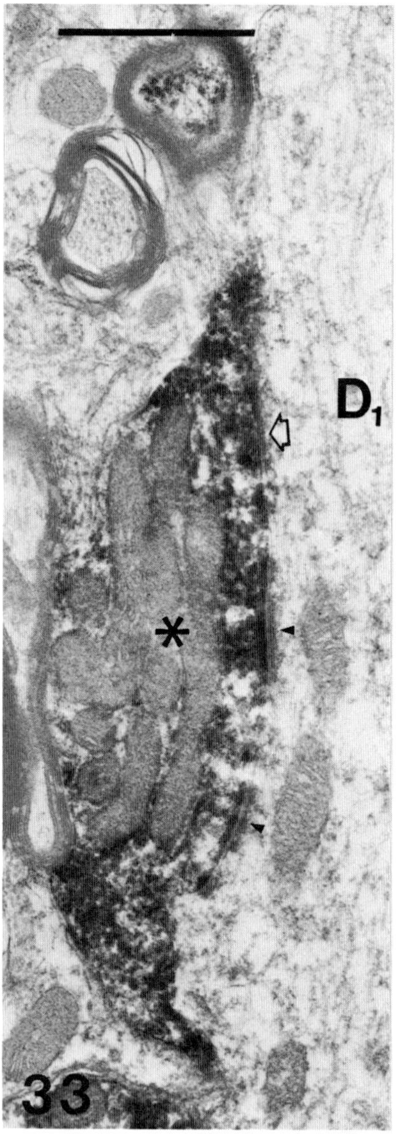

Fig. 32. Example of a pallidal bouton (PT) in the VA labeled after injection of tritiated leucine in the entopeduncular nucleus of the cat. Open arrows point to symmetrical synapses between the PT and a primary dendrite of TCPN (D_1). Bar = 1 μm. Modified from Kultas-Ilinsky et al. [105].

Fig. 33. An axon terminal (asterisk) in the VA displaying positive immunoreactivity with antibody to GAD. An open arrow points to symmetrical synapse between the bouton and a primary dendrite of TCPN (D_1). Small arrowheads point to puncta adherentes. Bar = 1 μm. Modified from Kultas-Ilinsky et al. [78].

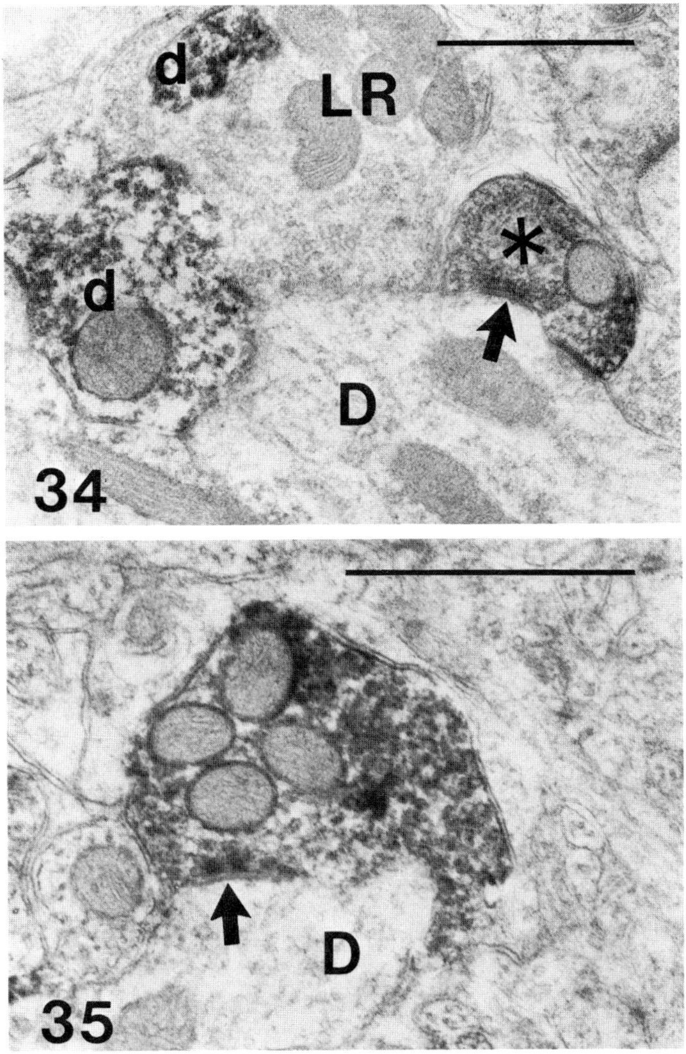

Figs. 34, 35. Examples of GAD-positive boutons in the cat VL (arrows). A small terminal indicated by an asterisk in Fig. 34, and the bouton demonstrated in Fig. 35 most likely correspond to F3 and F2 terminals, respectively [9]. D, TCPN dendrites; d, GAD-positive LCN dendrites; LR, LR bouton. Bars = 1 μ. From Kultas-Ilinsky et al. [78], with permission.

description and the illustrations provided they were identical to the terminals of cortical afferents. One can assume that a massive involvement in the lesion of corticothalamic fibers in the internal capsule was responsible for a large number of the cortical type of degenerating boutons observed in this study, although the authors presented neither a description nor documentation of their lesions. Another reason for these findings, which contradict all other data, may be that the samples for EM analysis in experiments with pallidal lesions were taken from nuclear subdivisions with sparse or no pallidal input. The latter explanation appears very likely, considering one exception to their findings–namely, that in two tissue blocks from "a restricted-VL region" degenerating boutons similar to LR-type terminals were observed and interpreted as being of cerebellar origin, in spite of the fact that no cerebellar lesions were done in these experiments. The ease with which pallidal boutons can be mistaken for LR terminals has already been mentioned. As the data in the cat demonstrate, some of the pallidal boutons can be very large [105], and the synaptic vesicle morphology is substantially distorted even at early degeneration stages. Thus, it is not possible to determine their true size and shape and apply it for identification.

The findings on the ultrastructure of pallidal afferents in the cat obtained in different laboratories and with different techniques are consistent and are partially confirmed by findings in the squirrel monkey [135]. In addition, the physiological data [68,69,71,72] on the inhibitory nature of this input, both in cat and monkey, correlate with the morphology of these boutons (pleomorphic vesicles, symmetrical contacts) and therefore challenge the results of Harding and Powell [6] in regard to this system. Further studies using other experimental techniques available at present are needed to verify the termination sites and the specific morphology of pallidal afferents in primates.

Nigral terminals in the motor thalamus have been identified by degeneration and EM autoradiography (Fig. 21) only in the cat [28,35,105]. In the degeneration study that used electrolytic lesions in the SNr they were found to display features of electron-dense degeneration [35]. However, we have recently found (Kultas-Ilinsky and Ilinsky, unpublished) that nigral boutons can display features of both electron-dense and electron-lucent types of degeneration after lesions induced by neurotoxic amino acids (Figs. 30, 31). The earlier degeneration study [35] showed the nigral boutons to be of medium size, to contain pleomorphic vesicles, and to form symmetrical contacts. In other words, they were basically similar to pallidal terminals, except that nigral afferents formed exclusively "bouton terminaux"type endings. In a recent EM autoradiography study [105] it was shown that the average size of nigral boutons was larger than that antici-

TABLE II. Distribution of synaptic sites of nigral and pallidal afferents

Postsynaptic structure	% of boutons in contact with each postsynaptic structure Pallidal (N = 100)	Nigral (N = 100)
Somata of thalamocortical projection neurons (TCPN)	21	0
(Percentage of the above at the bases of primary dendrites)	(66)	0
Primary TCPN dendrites	19	28.8
(Percentage of the above at the bifurcation of primary dendrites)	(37)	(49)
Secondary TCPN dendrites	36	30.6
(Percentage of the above at the bifurcation of secondary dendrites)	(9)	(4)
Tertiary TCPN dendrites	13	23.6
Dendrites of local-circuit neurons	8.0	8.2
Unidentified	3.0	8.8

From Kultas-Ilinsky et al. [105], with permission.

pated from degeneration studies [35]. The earlier underestimation of the size of boutons apparently resulted from degeneration-induced shrinkage of the terminals.

Comparison of qualitative and quantitative features of nigral and pallidal terminals in an EM autoradiography study failed to reveal any significant differences in the size or shape of synaptic vesicles or any other characteristics [105]. Thus, both terminals were classified as MP-type boutons, described earlier in the normal neuropil of VM (see Section 5.1). Although both inputs are directed mainly to primary and secondary dendrites of TCPN and show a tendency to be located at their bifurcation sites, the synaptic sites of the nigral terminals differed from those of the pallidal terminals. Nigral boutons were less often found on somata of TCPN and more frequently on their tertiary dendrites (Table II). Additionally, labeled nigral boutons, unlike the pallidal, were observed in glomeruli. The inhibitory nature of the nigral input has been documented in numerous electrophysiological studies in different species [62,66,67,136,137]. The striking similarity in morphology of nigral and pallidal boutons is therefore not surprising. It is noteworthy that in the cat stimulation of the substantia nigra has been shown to result in a variety of responses by cells identified physiologically as TCPN. These include short-latency and long-latency inhibitions and polysynaptic long-latency excitation [136]. These findings correlate well with a variety of termination sites of the nigral boutons. More recently, an immunocytochemical study in the cat motor thalamus [78] has shown that synaptic terminals displaying features of both pallidal and nigral boutons are GAD-positive [Fig. 33] and are found in VM and VA but not in VL. This confirmed the earlier indirect evidence [137–139] in favor of GABA as the neurotransmitter of the basal ganglia input to the thalamus. Moreover, this study demonstrated the existence of contacts between the GAD-positive boutons and GAD-containing dendrites of LCN, thus providing an anatomical substrate for disinhibition in the motor thalamus. In the case of nigral afferents, such relationships may be responsible for the long-latency excitation observed in electrophysiological experiments [136].

5.2.5 Other afferent inputs. As noted earlier (see Section 3.4) little information is available on the topography of other afferents to the region suggested by light microscope studies, and nothing is known about the ultrastructural features of these putative afferents. In the studies discussed above on identification of the afferent origin of synaptic terminals, most types of boutons described in the normal neuropil of the motor thalamus have been accounted for, except for the F2 and F3 types of Rinvik and Grofová [9]. Interestingly, two types of GABAergic terminals that differed from the basal ganglia boutons were found in the VL [78], and these can be considered as the counterparts of the F2 and F3 boutons (Figs. 34, 35). However, comparison of the fine-structural features of these terminals in the normal neuropil with those in immunocytochemical preparations poses some difficulties owing to heavy deposits of reaction product that obscure some ultrastructural features. Since the VL lacks basal ganglia input, it has been suggested that the larger GAD-positive terminals in the VL, such as shown in Figure 35, may originate from the axons of the reticular thalamic nucleus. The cells in this nucleus show a strong GAD-positive reaction [140]; therefore their axon terminals can be expected to be GAD-positive also. This assumption was based on the similarity of these boutons to reticular terminals identified in other thalamic nuclei [141,142]. Until additional data are available, however, this must remain speculative same as another possibility that GABAergic F2 and F3 type boutons may represent the terminals of LCN axons.

6 SUMMARY OF SPECIFIC FEATURES OF SYNAPTIC ORGANIZATION IN INDIVIDUAL NUCLEAR SUBDIVISIONS OF THE MOTOR THALAMUS

From the above description it is clear that compared to other species the cat motor thalamus is best understood in regard to the relationships of different afferent systems on thalamic neurons. The question now is whether any synaptic patterns can be detected that are characteristic of individual nuclei, each of which receive specific combinations of afferents. There are no published data concerning this topic and, as mentioned earlier, in most studies on the synaptology of the motor thalamus this question was not addressed. In an attempt to throw light on this issue, we have recently begun a comparative quantitative analysis of normal synaptic organization of the individual motor thalamic nuclei in the cat. The motor thalamus was divided into three regions according to the major subcortical afferent inputs received by each: 1) VL, the thalamic area receiving mainly cerebellar afferents, 2) VA and anterolateral VM, the area of overlap of nigral and pallidal projections, and 3) medial VM, the thalamic area that receives its major input from the substantia nigra. EM specimens were obtained from each of these regions, and various quantitative and qualitative parameters of the synaptic organization of the neuropil are being compared. Although data are still preliminary, some clear trends can be mentioned in regard to the organization of synaptic inputs on TCPN in these subdivisions of the motor thalamus.

6.1 Synaptic Organization of the VL

The most typical feature of the VL neuropil is the presence of numerous glomeruli. According to our preliminary estimate they occupy at least 50% of the volume of the neuropil of the VL. Glomeruli in the VL are characterized by large numbers of LR boutons, whose cerebellar origin has previously been demonstrated (see Section 5.2.3). The major GABAergic profile in the VL glomeruli is represented by vesicle-containing dendrites of LCN [78].

Analysis of the extraglomerular neuropil of the VL shows that synaptic boutons on somata of TCPN are very few. When present, they are represented by medium-sized GABAergic axon terminals [78] that probably belong to the F2 type of Rinvik and Grofová [9] but are of unknown origin at present. Additonally, TCPN somata may receive symmetrical synapses from GABAergic LCN dendrites that are a part of serial synapses with SR-type boutons, although the final proof for this relationship is yet to be obtained.

Primary dendrites of TCPN can be roughly divided into two categories based on the density of synaptic coverage. Some of them appear to receive very few or no synaptic contacts, whereas moderate quantities of terminals can be seen on others (Fig. 36). In the latter an average of 8–30% of total membrane length is apposed by synaptic boutons. The boutons found on the primary dendrites are usually of the LR type, whose cerebellar origin has been verified [128]; only occasionally are F-type terminals of unidentified origin seen at these sites. This relationship results

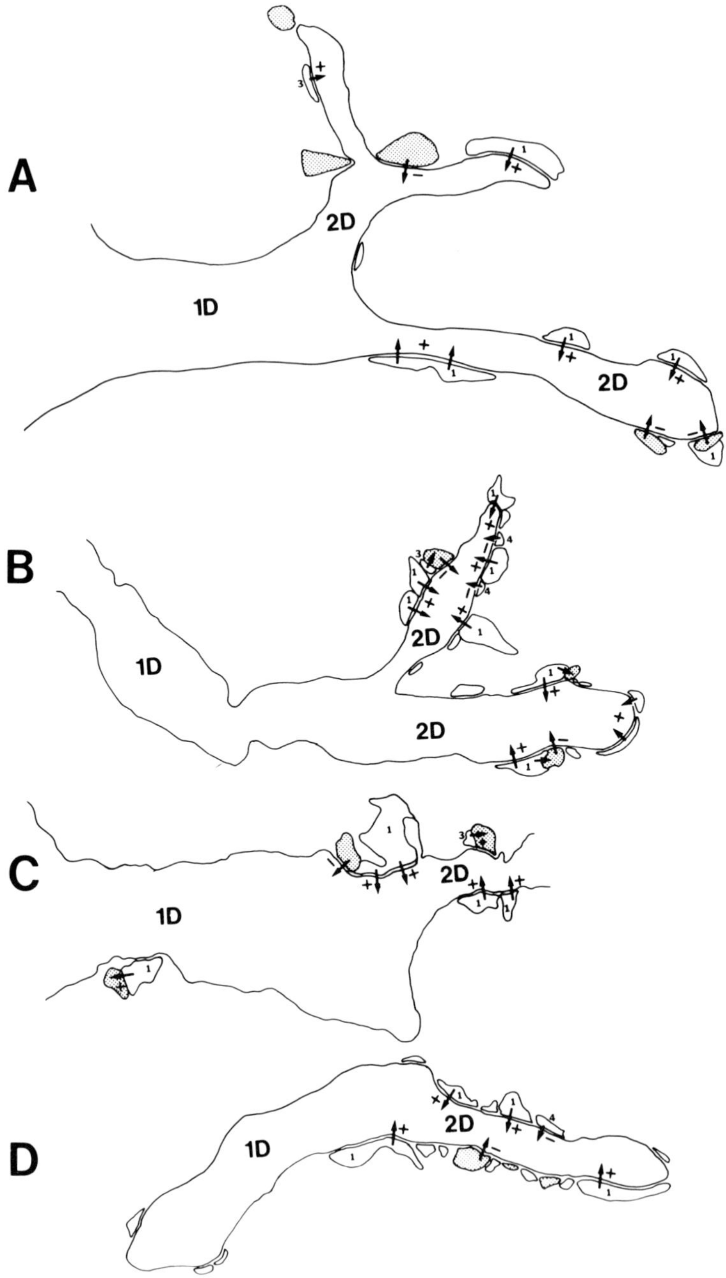

Fig. 36. Tracings of typical dendrites and associated structures from electron micrographs of the VL neuropil (A–D). Note absence of synaptic boutons on some primary (1D) dendrites (A,B) and the dense synaptic coverage on secondary (2D) dendrites (B and D). Note also the presence of complex synaptic arrangements, such as triads and serial synapses. Vesicle-containing dendrites of LCN are shown as shadowed profiles; small numerals mark different-type synaptic boutons: 1, LR-type boutons; 3, SR-type boutons; 4, F-type boutons of unknown origin. The sites and direction of synaptic contacts are indicated by arrows. + indicates asymmetrical contact; − indicates symmetrical contact.

in a relatively high (70%) proportion of asymmetric synaptic contacts on primary dendrites in the VL. At bifurcation sites of primary dendrites LR terminals are seen very often in triads (Fig. 36C). Also, single dendrodendritic synapses are very frequently found at these sites (Fig. 36A). After the first bifurcation synaptic coverage of secondary branches increases significantly, and the average of the total membrane length occupied by synaptic boutons is approximately 54%. The predominant bouton type on secondary dendrites is again the LR terminal, although a significant number of small-sized boutons with characteristic features of the F3 type of Rinvik and Grofová [9] are also present. SR boutons on secondary dendrites are encountered rarely, whereas dendrodendritic synapses are extremely frequent and the majority of them form a part of triads with LR boutons or serial synapses with SR boutons (Fig. 36). On tertiary branches 90% of the terminals are represented by SR boutons of cortical origin, and the overall density of synapses on these dendrites is relatively high (mean 80% of membrane apposed by synaptic boutons).

Summarizing the above data on the organization of synaptic inputs on the TCPN dendrites in the VL, one can say that most of the afferent input is directed towards secondary and tertiary dendrites and glomeruli, only a minor amount being received by somata and primary dendrites. As mentioned earlier (Section 5), there is a good correlation between anatomical and physiological studies on the motor thalamus in that the terminals of identified afferent systems with asymmetrical synaptic contacts have been shown to be excitatory and those with symmetrical contacts inhibitory. If we assume that these anatomical-physiological correlates are valid for all types of boutons in the motor thalamus, our data on the frequency of different types of synaptic boutons on the TCPN dendrites indicate that the excitatory input to the VL cells (LR and SR boutons) predominates. Based on the results of EM autoradiography and degeneration studies, the excitatory input arrives from two major sources, cerebellum and cortex. The inhibition to TCPN dendrites in the VL is provided by three types of contacts: dendrodendritic synapses and those formed by two types of F terminals of unidentified origin, all of which are GABAergic according to immunocytochemical evidence [78]. The dendrodendritic contacts outnumber those formed by F terminals, occupy a strategic location on TCPN dendrites, and mediate the indirect input from SR and LR type terminals.

6.2 Synaptic Organization of the VA and Anterolateral VM

Unlike the VL, glomeruli in this subdivision as well as in the medial VM are significantly less frequent, so that most of the neuropil is represented by the extraglomerular compartment. The glomeruli in this region differ from those in VL as well as from those in all other thalamic nuclei, since in addition to regular components they contain medium- to large-sized GAD-positive boutons of nigral origin (Section 5.1).

In addition various aspects of synaptic organization of extraglomerular neuropil in this region appear to be quite different from those in the VL. Although the serial synapses with SR boutons and GABAergic LCN dendrites are present on somata of TCPN, they are outnumbered by basal ganglia terminals which form symmetrical axosomatic synapses and are sometimes found in pairs on the perikarya of projection neurons. These boutons have been shown to be mainly of pallidal origin [105] and are GABAergic [78].

Primary dendrites of TCPN can also be subdivided into two categories: those that do not appear to receive any synapses, and others that have a moderate coverage by synaptic boutons (mean 17% of membrane occupied). Unlike VL, however, the terminals found on the second category of dendrites are represented exclusively by basal ganglia boutons forming symmetrical contacts. These are located at the bases of primary dendrites along the dendritic shafts and are grouped around the first bifurcation site. Even on those primary dendrites that do not bear axon terminals on their more proximal parts (i.e., type I dendrites), several basal ganglia type boutons are usually found at the first branching site.

Secondary dendrites in this region also differ according to the density of terminals on them. On some dendrites up to 50% of membrane length is apposed by synaptic boutons, whereas others seem not to receive any synapses. Thus, in general, synaptic coverage of secondary dendrites in this region is much lower than that in the VL. Another difference is that about 75% of the boutons on secondary dendrites display features of basal ganglia boutons (i.e., MP type—pleomorphic vesicles, symmetrical contacts, etc.), whereas the rest are mainly of the LR type. As in the VL, SR-type boutons when present on secondary dendrites are mainly a component of serial synapses. Dendrodendritic synapses on secondary dendrites are much less frequent than in the VL, and on those dendrites that have large numbers of basal ganglia boutons the dendrodendritic contacts are relatively rare. In general dendrodendritic contacts and basal ganglia terminals appear to be mutually exclusive. The synaptic coverage on secondary dendrites usually increases at the distal bifurcation. At this location, in addition to basal ganglia boutons, some LR terminals in triads are present. Such triads are also numerous on some tertiary branches, whereas on other tertiary branches SR boutons prevail (Fig. 37).

Thus, in this region of the motor thalamus the secondary and tertiary dendritic branches of TCPN vary significantly regarding combinations of types of synaptic boutons associated with them. This is different from the VL, where these combinations are similar and are typical for all dendrites of each particular order. When the quantitative analysis is completed, we expect that the data will provide information on the ratio of dendrites with

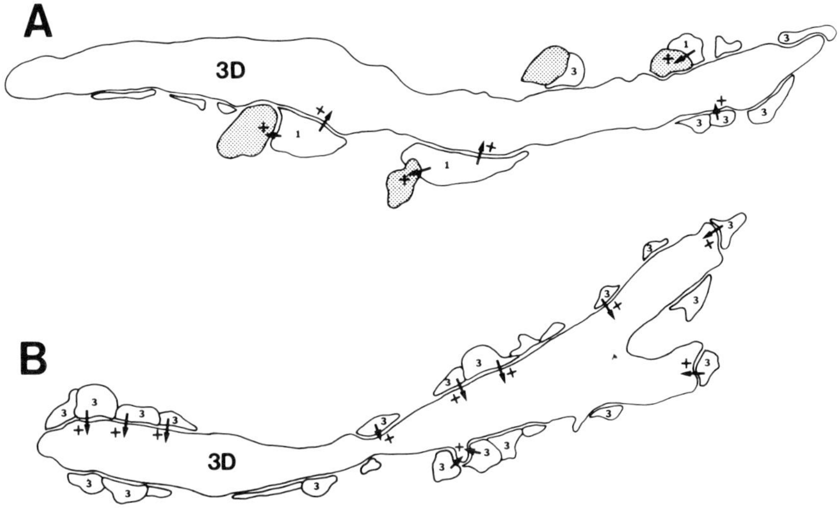

Fig. 37. Two variants of tertiary dendrites (3D) observed in the VA and anterolateral VM. Note the high density of SR boutons on dendrite B and prevalence of LR boutons on dendrite A, as in Figure 36.

different patterns of synaptic coverage. However, until studies specifically aimed at this question are available, it will remain unclear whether the dendrites with diverse synaptic patterns originate from the same or from different parent cells.

Summarizing the above data concerning the extraglomerular neuropil of the VA and anterolateral VM, it appears that the afferent input to proximal parts of TCPN (soma, primary, and secondary dendrites) is sparse, mainly inhibitory, and derived primarily from basal ganglia afferents and to a much lesser extent from GABAergic dendrites of LCN. Most of the excitatory input (SR and LR boutons) is directed to tertiary dendritic branches. Thus, the organization is essentially different from that in the VL, where such heavy extrinsic inhibitory input is absent. Our observations also indicate that the proportion of LR boutons in the neuropil of anterolateral VM and VA is relatively low compared to that in the VL neuropil. Therefore, it appears that the major excitatory input to confront the basal ganglia-derived inhibition should be mainly from SR terminals, i.e. cortical afferents.

6.3 Synaptic Organization of Medial VM

In a GAD immunocytochemical study [78] it was noted that the medial part of the VM differs from the VA and anterolateral VM by a

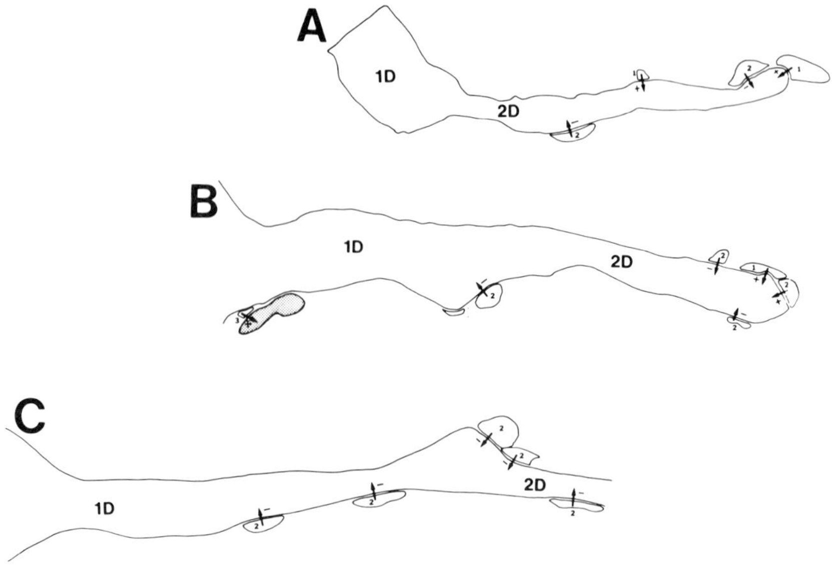

Fig. 38. Typical examples (A–C) of primary and secondary dendrites in the medial VM. Small numeral (2) marks MP type boutons. Labeling as in Figure 36.

lower density of GAD-positive terminals with features of basal ganglia boutons. This is especially true in regard to somata of TCPN, where such boutons are infrequent. On secondary and tertiary dendrites these boutons are present but they are more dispersed than at similar sites in the VA. In addition to serial synapses with SR boutons on TCPN somata, GAD-containing boutons with features different from those of boutons of basal ganglia origin were observed in the medial VM [78]. This suggests that the input to the perikarya of TCPN in the VA and anterolateral VM may be derived from a source different from that in the medial VM. Synaptic coverage of primary dendrites in the medial VM (Fig. 38) is variable, as it is in the VL and VA. In those instances where synaptic boutons are present, they appose up to 20% of the dendritic membrane. In all instances these terminals have features of basal ganglia boutons, which are concentrated at bifurcation sites of primary dendrites. However, unlike the VA and anterolateral VM, some LR boutons in triads may also be present at these bifurcation sites. On secondary dendrites synaptic coverage is higher than on primary branches, adding up on average to about 30% of membrane apposed by boutons. Differences between individual dendritic branches regarding the combinations of synaptic boutons that synapse upon them have been also noted in this subdivision. For example, on some secondary dendrites in the medial VM, the proportion of LR and SR boutons and the number of dendrodendritic contacts is high, whereas on others only basal ganglia boutons are present. On tertiary dendrites the general features of the arrangement and density of synaptic terminals is similar to that in the VA and anterolateral region of the VM. In general, compared to the latter areas, the region of the medial VM displays more diversity in synaptic patterns on different-order dendritic branches of TCPN.

Thus the main differences between the two regions (medial VM as opposed to VA and anterolateral VM) appear to be the lower density of basal ganglia boutons and the moderately high frequency of terminals with asymmetrical contacts (LR and SR) on secondary TCPN dendrites in the medial VM. This suggests that the ratio of inhibitory to excitatory inputs in this nucleus is roughly equal, unlike that in the VA and anterolateral VM.

6.4 General Comments

The description of synaptic patterns in individual subdivisions of the cat motor thalamus given above shows that differences can be detected in regard to quantitative aspects of synaptic relationships on TCPN dendrites. In some cases (VL versus VA, for example) these differences are obvious; in others (VA versus medial VM) they are more subtle and can be brought out only by tedious quantitative analysis of statistically large samples. The most notable difference between VL on the one hand, and VA and VM on the other, concerns the organization of inhibitory circuits. This was noted earlier in an immunocytochemical study [78], and a similar picture emerges from analysis of the normal neuropil. The data suggest that the dendrodendritic contacts formed by LCNs play a major role in inhibitory circuits in the VL, whereas in the VA and to some extent in the medial VM their role appears to be secondary to a heavy inhibitory input from the basal ganglia. In this respect the ultrastructure of the VL is more like that of other relay nuclei of the thalamus, whereas very little similarity between the latter and the VA and VM can be detected. In these two subdivisions the scarcity of excitatory terminals on primary and secondary TCPN dendrites is a characteristic feature, and it raises a question about the identity of the main driving force for these cells.

In conclusion, the anatomical data clearly demonstrate that there are significant differences in synaptic organization between individual subdivisions of the cat motor thalamus and that these correlate well with differences in the combinations of afferent inputs received by each region. Moreover, the data suggest that the inputs from a single afferent system may be organized differently in individual subdivisions, but a great deal has to be learned before the specifics of synaptic organization of each region are entirely understood. One can also predict that when similar studies become available in regard to the primate motor thalamus, they will show that the differences in synaptic organization between individual subdivisions in this case are even more pronounced than in the cat. The tendency towards segregation of inputs to separate neuronal populations, and therefore probably narrower specialization of each subset of nerve cells in the motor thalamus in phylogeny supports this assumption.

7 ACKNOWLEDGMENTS

This work was made possible by National Institutes of Health grants NS R0119280 and NSRR01171 and by grants from The American Parkinson Disease Association. We would like also to thank Brenda Robinson for assistance with art work and Tena Perry, Becky Stumpf, and Jo Ann Barnes for secretarial assistance.

8 REFERENCES

1. Jones EG: Functional subdivision and synaptic organization of the mammalian thalamus. In Porter T (ed): "International Review of Physiology." Baltimore: University Park Press, 1981, Vol 25, pp 173–245.
2. Grofová I, Rinvik E: Cortical and pallidal projections of the nucleus ventralis lateralis thalami. Electron microscopical studies in the cat. Anat Embryol 146:113–132, 1974.
3. Harding BN: Dendro-dendritic synapses, including reciprocal synapses, in the ventrolateral nucleus of the monkey thalamus. Brain Res 34:181–185, 1971.
4. Harding BN: An ultrastructural study of the termination of afferent fibres within the ventrolateral and centre median nuclei of the monkey thalamus. Brain Res 54:341–346, 1973.
5. Harding BN: An ultrastructural study of the centre median and ventrolateral thalamic nuclei of the monkey. Brain Res 54:335–340, 1973.
6. Harding BN, Powell TPS: An electron microscopic study of the centre-median and ventrolateral nuclei of the thalamus in the monkey. Phil Trans R Soc Lond (Biol) 279:357–412, 1977.
7. Kiss A, Tömböl T: Golgi analysis and degeneration studies of the nucleus ventralis lateralis and ventralis medialis in the cat thalamus. Brain Res 47:303–315, 1972.
8. Pappas GD, Cohen, EB, Purpura DP: Fine structure of synaptic and nonsynaptic neuronal relations in the thalamus of the cat. In Purpura DP, Yahr MD (eds): "The Thalamus." New York: Columbia University Press, 1966, pp 47–71.
9. Rinvik E, Grofová I: Light and electron microscopical studies of the normal nuclei ventralis lateralis and ventralis anterior thalami in the cat. Anat Embryol 146:57–93, 1974.
10. Rinvik E, Grofová I: Cerebellar projections to the nucleus ventralis lateralis and ventralis anterior thalami. Anat Embryol 146:95–111, 1974.
11. Scheibel ME, Scheibel AB: The organization of the ventral anterior nucleus of the thalamus. A Golgi study. Brain Res 1:250–268, 1966.
12. Angaut P, Bowsher D: Ascending projections of the medial cerebellar (fastigial) nucleus: An experimental study in the cat. Brain Res 24:49–68, 1970.
13. Angaut P: The ascending projections of the nucleus interpositus posterior of the cat cerebellum: An experimental anatomical study using silver impregnation methods. Brain Res 24:337–394, 1970.
14. Asanuma C, Thach WT, Jones EG: Distribution of cerebellar terminations and their

relation to other afferent terminations in the ventral lateral thalamic region of the monkey. Brain Res Rev 5:237–265, 1983.
15. Asanuma C, Thach WT, Jones EG: Cytoarchitectonic delineation of the ventral lateral thalamic region in the monkey. Brain Res Rev 5:219–235, 1983.
16. Burton H, Craig AD: Spinothalamic projections in cat, racoon and monkey: A study based on anterograde transport of horseradish peroxidase. In Macchi G, Rustioni A, Spreafico R (eds): "Somatosensory Integration in the Thalamus." Amsterdam: Elsevier, 1983, pp 17–41.
17. Carpenter MB, Peter PH: Nigrostriatal and nigrothalamic fibers in the Rhesus monkey. J Comp Neurol 144:93–116, 1972.
18. Carpenter MB, Nakano K, Kim R: Nigrothalamic projections in the monkey demonstrated by autoradiographic technics. J Comp Neurol 165:401–416, 1976.
19. Carter DA, Fibiger HC: The projections of the entopeduncular nucleus and globus pallidus in rat as demonstrated by autoradiography and horseradish peroxidase histochemistry. J Comp Neurol 177:113–124, 1978.
20. Chan-Palay V: "Cerebellar Dentate Nucleus: Organization, Cytology and Transmitters." Berlin, Heidelberg, New York: Springer, 1977.
21. Clavier RM, Atmadja S, Fibiger HC: Nigrothalamic projections in the rat as demonstrated by orthograde and retrograde tracing techniques. Brain Res Bull 1:379–384, 1976.
22. DeVito JL, Anderson ME: An autoradiographic study of efferent connections of the globus pallidus in Macaca mulatta. Exp Brain Res 46:107–117, 1982.
23. Faull RLM, Carman JB: Ascending projections of the substantia nigra in the rat. J Comp Neurol 132:73–92, 1968.
24. Faull RLM, Carman JB: The cerebellofugal projections in the brachium conjunctivum of the rat. J Comp Neurol 178:495–518, 1978.
25. Haroian AJ, Massopust LC, Young PA: Cerebellothalamic projections in the rat: An autoradiographic and degeneration study. J Comp Neurol 197:217–236, 1981.
26. Hendry SHC, Jones EG, Graham J: Thalamic relay nuclei for cerebellar and certain related fiber systems in the cat. J Comp Neurol 185:679–714, 1979.
27. Herkenham M: The afferent and efferent connections of the ventromedial thalamic nucleus in the rat. J Comp Neurol 183:487–519, 1979.
28. Ilinsky IA, Kultas-Illinsky K, Smith KR: Organization of basal ganglia inputs to the thalamus. A light and electron microscopic study in the cat. Appl Neurophysiol 45:230–237, 1982.
29. Ilinsky IA, Kultas-Ilinsky K: An autoradiographic study of the topographical relationships between the pallidal and cerebellar projections to the cat thalamus. Exp Brain Res 54:95–106, 1984.
30. Ilinsky IA, Kultas-Ilinsky K: An autoradiographic study on organization of basal ganglia projections to the thalamus in the Rhesus monkey. Anat Rec 208:78, 1984.
31. Ilinsky IA, Jouandet ML, Goldman-Rakic PS: Organization of the nigrothalamocortical system in the Rhesus monkey. J Comp Neurol 236:315–330, 1985.
32. Kalil K: Projections of the cerebellar and dorsal column nuclei upon the thalamus of the Rhesus monkey. J Comp Neurol 195:25–50, 1981.
33. Kievet J, Kuypers HGJM: Organization of the thalamocortical connections to the frontal lobe in the Rhesus monkey. Exp Brain Res 29:299–322, 1977.
34. Kim R, Nakano K, Jayaraman A, Carpenter MB: Projections of the globus pallidus and adjacent structures: An autoradiographic study in the monkey. J Comp Neurol 169:263–290, 1976.
35. Kultas-Ilinsky K, Ilinsky IA, Massopust LC. Young PA, Smith KR: Nigrothalamic pathway in the cat demonstrated by autoradiography and electron-microscopy. Exp Brain Res 33:481–492, 1978.

36. Larsen DK, McBride RL: The organization of feline entopeduncular nucleus projections: Anatomical studies. J Comp Neurol 184:293–308, 1979.
37. Nauta HJW: Projections of the pallidal complex: An autoradiographic study in the cat. Neuroscience 4:1853–1873, 1979.
38. Percheron G: The thalamic territory of cerebellar afferents and the lateral region of the thalamus of the macaque in stereotaxic ventricular coordinates. J Hirnforsch 18:375–400, 1977,
39. Sugimoto T, Mizuno N, Itoh K: An autoradiographic study on the terminal distribution of cerebellothalamic fibers in the cat. Brain Res 215:29–47, 1981.
40. Tracey DJ, Asanuma C, Jones EG, Porter R: Thalamic relay to motor cortex: Efferent pathways from brain stem, cerebellum and spinal cord in monkeys. J Neurophysiol 44:532–554, 1980.
41. Clark WE, LeGros: The structure and connections of the thalamus. Brain 55:406–470, 1936.
42. Crouch RL: The nuclear configuration of the thalamus of Macacus Rhesus. J Comp Neurol 59:451–485, 1934.
43. Hassler R: Anatomy of the thalamus. In Schaltenbrand G, Bailey P (eds): "Introduction to Stereotaxic Operations with an Atlas of the Human Brain." Stuttgart: Thieme, 1959, pp 230–290.
44. Vogt G: La myéloarchitecture du thalamus de cercopithèque. J Psychol Neurol 12:285–324, 1909.
45. Olszewski J: The thalamus of Macaca mulatta. An atlas for use with the stereotaxic instrument. Basel: Karger, 1952.
46. Rinvik E: A re-evaluation of the cytoarchitecture of the ventral nuclear complex of the cat's thalamus on the basis of corticothalamic connections. Brain Res 8:237–254, 1968.
47. Berman AL, Jones EG: The thalamus and basal telencephalon of the cat. A cytoarchitectonic atlas with stereotaxic coordinates. Madison: University of Wisconsin Press, 1982.
48. Jasper H, Ajmone-Marson C: "A Stereotaxic Atlas of the Diencephalon of the Cat." Ottawa: University of Toronto Press, 1954.
49. Reinoso-Suárez F: "Topographischer Hirnatlas de Katze für experimental-physiologische Untersuchungen." Darmstadt: E Merck, 1961.
50. Jones EG, Burton H. Cytoarchitecture and somatic sensory connectivity of thalamic nuclei other than the ventrobasal complex in the cat. J Comp Neurol 154:395–432, 1974.
51. Beckstead RM, Domesick VB, Nauta WKH: Efferent connections of the substantia nigra and ventral tegmental area in the rat. Brain Res 175:191–217, 1979.
52. Stanton GB: Topographical organization of ascending cerebellar projections from the dentate and interposed nuclei in Macaca mulatta: An anterograde degeneration study. J Comp Neurol 190:699–731, 1980.
53. Rispal-Padel L, Grangetto A: The cerebello-thalamo-cortical pathway. Topographical investigation at the unitary level in the cat. Exp Brain Res 28:101–123, 1977.
54. Strick PL: Light microscopic analysis of the cortical projection of the thalamic ventral lateral nucleus in the cat. Brain Res 55:1–24, 1973.
55. Bentivoglio M, Macchi G, Rossini P, Tempesta E: Le proiezioni talamo-corticali del nucleo ventrale anteriore: studio mediante il transporto assonale retrogrado di HRP nel gatto. Arch Ital Anat Embryol 83:111–127, 1978.
56. Glenn LL, Hada J, Roy JP, Deschênes M, Steriade M: Anterograde tracers and field potential analysis of the neocortical layers. I. Projection from nucleus ventralis medialis of the thalamus in cat. Neuroscience 7:1861–1877, 1982.

57. Minciacchi D, Bentivoglio M, Molinari M, Kultas-Ilinsky K, Ilinsky I, Macchi G: Multiple cortical targets of one thalamic nucleus: The projections of the ventral medial nucleus in the cat studied with retrograde tracers. J Comp Neurol, in press.
58. Niimi K, Niimi M, Okada Y: Thalamic afferents to the limbic cortex in the cat studied with the method of retrograde axonal transport of horseradish peroxidase. Brain Res 145:225–238, 1978.
59. Roda JM, Reinoso-Suárez F: Topographic organization of the thalamic projections to the cortex of the anterior ectosylvian sulcus in the cat. Exp Brain Res 49:131–139, 1983.
60. Schell GR, Strick PL: Origin of thalamic input to the arcuate premotor and supplementary motor areas. J Neurosci 4:539–560, 1984.
61. Rinvik E: The corticothalamic projection from the pericruciate and coronal gyri in the cat. An experimental study with silver-impregnation methods. Brain Res 10:79–119, 1968.
62. Chevalier G, Deniau JM: Inhibitory nigral influence on cerebellar evoked responses in the rat ventromedial thalamic nucleus. Exp Brain Res 48:369–376, 1982.
63. James TA, MacLeod NK, Starr MS: The cerebello-thalamic pathway in the rat. J Physiol 313:29, 1980.
64. James TA, MacLeod NK: Regulation of the cerebello-thalamic relay in the rat. J Physiol 315:31, 1981.
65. MacLeod NK, James TA: Regulation of cerebello-cortical transmission in the rat ventromedial thalamic nucleus. Exp Brain Res 55:535–552, 1984.
66. Ueki A: The mode of nigro-thalamic transmission investigated with intracellular recording in the cat. Exp Brain Res 49:116–124, 1983.
67. Ueki A. Uno M, Anderson M, Yoshida M: Monosynaptic inhibition of thalamic neurons produced by stimulation of the substantia nigra. Experientia 33:1480–1481, 1977.
68. Uno M, Yoshida M: Monosynaptic inhibition of thalamic neurons produced by stimulation of the pallidal nucleus in cats. Brain Res 99:377–380, 1975.
69. Uno M, Ozawa N, Yoshida M: The mode of pallido-thalamic transmission investigated with intracellular recording from cat thalamus. Exp Brain Res 33:493–507, 1978.
70. Uno M, Yoshida M, Hirota I: The mode of cerebello-thalamic relay transmission investigated with intracellular recording from cells of the ventrolateral nucleus of cat's thalamus. Exp Brain Res 10:121–139, 1970.
71. Huffman RD, Felpel LP, Lum J: An extracellular microelectrode study of globus pallidus and cerebellar projections to the thalamus in the monkey. Soc Neurosci Abstr 10:180, 1984.
72. Yamamoto T, Hassler R, Huber C, Wagner A, Sasaki K: Electrophysiological studies of the pallido- and cerebellothalamic projections in Squirrel monkeys (Saimiri sciureus). Exp Brain Res 51:77–87, 1983.
73. Steriade M, Deschênes M: The thalamus as a neuronal oscillator. Brain Res Rev 8:1–63, 1984.
74. Scheibel ME, Scheibel AB: The organization of the nucleus reticularis thalami: A Golgi Study. Brain Res. 1:43–62, 1966.
75. Jones EG: Some aspects of the organization of the thalamic reticular complex. J Comp Neurol 162:285–308, 1975.
76. Herkenham M, Gerfen CR: An anterograde tracing study of the connections of the thalamic reticular nucleus in the rat. Anat Rec 211:82, 1985.
77. Steriade M, Parent A, Hada J: Thalamic projections of nucleus reticularis thalami of cat: A study using retrograde transport of horseradish peroxidase and fluorescent

tracers. J Comp Neurol 229:531–547, 1984.
78. Kultas-Ilinsky K, Ribak CE, Peterson GM, Oertel WH: A description of the GABA-ergic neurons and axon terminals in the motor nuclei of the cat thalamus. J Neurosci 5:1346–1369, 1985.
79. Harting JK, Huerta MF, Frankfurter AJ, Strominger NL, Royce GJ: Ascending pathways from the monkey superior colliculus: An autoradiographic analysis. J Comp Neurol 192:853–882, 1980.
80. Purpura DP, Frigyesi TL, McMurtry JG, Scarff T: Synaptic mechanisms in thalamic regulation of cerebello-cortical projection activity. In Purpura DP, Yahr MD (eds): "The Thalamus." New York: Columbia University Press, 1966, pp 153–172.
81. Robertson RT, Lynch GS, Thompson RF: Diencephalic distributions of ascending reticular systems. Brain Res 55:309–322, 1973.
82. Robertson RT, Feiner AL: Diencephalic projections from the pontine reticular formation: Autoradiographic studies in the cat. Brain Res 239:3–16, 1982.
83. Kultas-Ilinsky K, Warton S, Ilinsky IA: Light and electron microscopical features of two types of neurons in the cat's ventral medial thalamic nucleus as revealed with HRP injections in the motor cortex. Soc Neurosci Abstr 7:416, 1981.
84. White EL, Hersch SM, Rock MP: Synaptic sequences in mouse SmI cortex involving pyramidal cells labeled by retrograde filling with horseradish peroxidase. Neurosci Lett 19:149–154, 1980.
85. Al-Hussain S, Kultas-Ilinsky K: Geometry and quantitative characteristics of dendritic arbors of thalamocortical projection neurons in the cat VA and VM. Soc Neurosci Abstr 11:678, 1985.
86. Dodge, FA: The nonuniform excitability of central neurons as exemplified by a model of the spinal motoneuron. In Schmitt FO, Worden FG (eds): "The Neurosciences Fourth Study Program." Cambridge: MIT Press, 1979, pp 439–455.
87. Hillman DE: Neuronal shape parameters and substructures as a basis of neuronal form. In Schmitt FO, Worden FG (eds): "The Neurosciences Fourth Study Program." Cambridge: MIT Press, 1979, pp 477–498.
88. Yamamoto T, Noda T, Samejima A, Oka H: A morphological investigation of thalamic neurons by intracellular HRP staining in cats. J Comp Neurol 236:331–347, 1985.
89. Tsukahara N: Synaptic plasticity in the red nucleus. In Cotman CW (ed): "Neuronal Plasticity." New York: Raven, 1978, pp 335–348.
90. Tömböl T: Short neurons and their synaptic relations in the specific thalamic nuclei. Brain Res 3:307–326, 1967.
91. Famiglietti EV, Peters A: The synaptic glomerulus and the intrinsic neuron in the dorsal lateral geniculate nucleus of the cat. J Comp Neurol 114:285–334, 1972.
92. LeVay S: On the neurons and synapses of the lateral geniculate nucleus of the monkey and the effects of eye enucleation. Z Zellforsch 113:396–419, 1971.
93. Lieberman AR: Neurons with presynaptic perikarya and presynaptic dendrites in the rat lateral geniculate nucleus. Brain Res 59:35–59, 1973.
94. Beckstead RM: The thalamostriatal projection in the cat. J Comp Neurol 223:313–346, 1984.
95. Macchi G, Bentivoglio M, Molinari M, Minciacchi D: The thalamo-caudate versus thalamo-cortical projections as studied in the cat with fluorescent retrograde double labeling. Exp Brain Res 54:225–239, 1984.
96. Royce, GJ: Cells of origin of subcortical afferents to the caudate nucleus: A horseradish peroxidase study in the cat. Brain Res 153:465–475, 1978.
97. Royce, GJ: Single thalamic neurons which project to both the rostral cortex and

caudate nucleus studied with the fluorescent double labeling method. Exp Neurol 79:773–784, 1983.

98. Scheibel ME, Scheibel AB: Structural organization of nonspecific thalamic nuclei and their projection toward cortex. Brain Res 6:60–94, 1967.
99. Kultas-Ilinsky K, Ilinsky IA, Young PA, Smith KR: Ultrastructure of degenerating cerebellothalamic terminals in the ventral medial nucleus of the cat. Exp Brain Res 38:125–135, 1980.
100. Penny, GR, Conley M, Diamond IT, Schmechel DE: A comparative study of the thalamic distribution of GAD immunoreactive neurons. Soc Neurosci Abstr 9:921, 1983.
101. Kultas-Ilinsky K, Ilinsky IA, Smith KR: Fine structure of the ventral medial thalamic nucleus in the cat. Anat Rec 193:594, 1979.
102. Jones EG, Powell TPS: Electron microscopy of synaptic glomeruli in the thalamic relay nuclei of the cat. Proc Roy Soc 172:153–171, 1969.
103. Morest DK: Synaptic relationships of Golgi Type II cells in the medial geniculate body of the cat. J Comp Neurol 162:157–194, 1975.
104. Ralston III JH: The synaptic organization of leminiscal projections to the ventrobasal thalamus of the cat. Brain Res 14:99–115, 1969.
105. Kultas-Ilinsky K, Ilinsky I, Warton S, Smith KR: Fine structure of nigral and pallidal afferents in the thalamus: An EM autoradiography study in the cat. J Comp Neurol 216:390–405, 1983.
106. Purpura DP: Synaptic mechanisms in coordination of activity in thalamic internuncial common path. In Frigyesi T, Rinvik E, Yahr MD (eds): "Corticothalamic Projections and Sensorimotor Activities." New York: Raven, 1972, pp 21–56.
107. Ralston III HJ: Neuronal circuitry of the ventrobasal thalamus: The role of presynaptic dendrites. In Schmitt FO, Worden FG (eds): "The Neurosciences Fourth Study Program." Cambridge: MIT Press, 1979, pp 373–379.
108. Pasik P, Pasik T, Hāmori J: Synapses between interneurons in the lateral geniculate nucleus of monkeys. Exp Brain Res 25:1–13, 1976.
109. Hámori J, Pasik P, Pasik T, Szentágothai J: Triadic synaptic arrangements and their possible significance in the lateral geniculate nucleus of the monkey. Brain Res 80:379–393, 1974.
110. Dekker JJ, Kuypers HGJM: Morphology of rat's AV thalamic nucleus in light and electron microscopy. Brain Res 177:387–398, 1976.
111. Garey LJ, Hornung JP: The use of ibotenic acid lesions for light and electron microscopic study of anterograde degeneration in the visual pathway of the cat. Neurosci Lett 19:117–123, 1980.
112. Olney JW: Kainic acid and other excitotoxins: A comparative analysis. In DiChiara G, Gesa GL (eds): "Glutamate as a Neurotransmitter." New York: Raven, 1981, pp 375–385.
113. Peterson GM, Moore RY: Selective effects of kainic acid on diencephalic neurons. Brain Res 200:165–182, 1980.
114. Schwarcz R, Coyle JT: Striatal lesions with kainic acid: Neurochemical characteristics. Brain Res 127:235–249, 1977.
115. Schwarcz R, Hökfelt T, Fuxe K, Jonsson G, Goldstein M, Terenius L: Ibotenic acid-induced neuronal degeneration: A morphological and neurochemical study. Exp Brain Res 37:199–215, 1979.
116. Sperk G, Lassman H, Baran H, Kish SJ, Seitelberger F, Hornykiewicz O: Kainic acid induced seizures: Neurochemical and histopathological changes. Neuroscience 10:1301–1315, 1983.

117. Wuerthele SM, Lovell KL, Jones MZ, Moore KE: A histological study of kainic acid-induced lesions in the rat brain. Brain Res 149:489–497, 1978.
118. Malmgren L, Olsson Y: A sensitive method for histochemical demonstration of horseradish peroxidase in neurons following retrograde axonal transport. Brain Res 148:279–294, 1978.
119. Kultas-Ilinsky K, Taylor J, Smith KR: Electron microscopy of corticothalamic degeneration in the rat. Anat Rec 184:454, 1976.
120. Jones EG, Powell TPS: An electron microscope study of the mode of termination of cortical thalamic fibers within the sensory relay nuclei of the thalamus. Proc Roy Soc 172:173–185, 1969.
121. Bava A, Circirata F, Licciardello S, Panto MR: Organizzazione delle proiezioni cortico-talamiche, originate dalle aree somatiche a motorici, su neuroni del nucleo di relais diencefalico della via cerebello-cerebrale (VL). Studio elettrofisiologico. Boll Soc Ital Biol Sper 56:1707–1714, 1980.
122. Frigyesi TL, Machek J: Basal ganglia-diencephalon synaptic relations in the cat. I. An intracellular study of dorsal thalamic neurons during capsular and basal ganglia stimulation. Brain Res 20:201–217, 1970.
123. Frigyesi TL, Schwartz R: Cortical control of thalamic sensorimotor relay activities in the cat and the squirrel monkey. In Frigyesi T, Rinvik, E, Yahr MD (eds): "Corticothalamic Projections and Sensorimotor Activities." New York: Raven, 1972, pp 161–191.
124. Roy JP, Clercq M, Steriade M, Deschênes M: Electrophysiology of neurons of the lateral thalamic nuclei in cat: Mechanisms of long-lasting hyper-polarizations. J Neurophysiol 51:1220–1235, 1984.
125. Fonnum F, Storm-Mathisen J, Divac I: Biochemical evidence for glutamate as a neurotransmitter in corticostriatal and corticothalamic fibres in the rat brain. Neuroscience 6:863–873, 1981.
126. Fonnum F, Soreide A, Kvale I, Walker J, Walaas I: Glutamate in cortical fibers. In DiChiara G, Gessa GL (eds): "Glutamate as a Neurotransmitter." New York: Raven, 1981, pp 29–41.
127. Young AB, Bromberg MB, Penney JB: Decreased glutamate uptake in subcortical areas deafferented by sensorimotor coritcal ablation in the cat. J Neurosci 1:241–249, 1981.
128. Kultas-Ilinsky K, Warton S, Tolbert DL, Ilinsky IA: Quantitative and qualitative characteristics of dentate and fastigial afferents identified by electron microscopic autoradiography in the cat thalamus. Brain Res 201:220–226, 1980.
129. Bava A, Circirata F, Licciardello S, LiVolsi G, Panto M: Fastigial nuclei projections on the ventralis lateralis (VL) thalamic nucleus neurons. Brain Res 168:169–175, 1979.
130. Matsuda Y, Nakamura M: Mode of activation of thalamic neurons by stimulation of the cerebellar fastigial nuclei in the cat. Brain Res 241:370–373, 1982.
131. Bava A, Circirata F, Licciardello S, Panto MR: Fenomeni di convergenza evocati in neuroni del nucleo ventralis lateralis del talamo (VL) dalla stimolazione di afferenze d'origine paleo- e neocerebellare. Boll Soc Ital Biol Sper 56:1693–1700, 1980.
132. Nieoullon A, Kerkerian L, Dusticier N: High affinity glutamate uptake in the red nucleus and ventrolateral thalamus after lesion of the cerebellum in adult cat. Exp Brain Res 55:409–419, 1984.
133. Marshall KC, Flumerfelt BA, Gwyn DG: Acetylcholinesterase activity and acetylcholine effects in the cerebello-rubro-thalamic pathway of the cat. Brain Res 190:493–504, 1980.

134. MacLeod NK, James TA, Starr MS: Muscarinic action of acetylcholine in the rat ventromedial thalamic nucleus. Exp Brain Res 55:553–561, 1984.
135. Nitecka L, Hassler, R, Bialowas J, Wagner A: The different types of synapses in the thalamic nucleus ventralis anterior (VA) of Saimiri sciureus and their degeneration after pallidum coagulation. J Hirnforsch 24:149–164, 1983.
136. Deniau JM, Lackner D, Feger J: Effect of substantia nigra stimulation on identified neurons in the VL-VA thalamic complex comparison between intact and chronically decorticated cats. Brain Res 145:27–35, 1978.
137. MacLeod NK, James TA, Kilpatrick IC, Starr MS: Evidence for a GABAergic nigrothalamic pathway in the rat. Exp Brain Res 40:55–61, 1980.
138. DiChiara G, Porceddu ML, Morelli M, Mulas ML, Gessa GL: Evidence for a GABA-ergic projection from the substantia nigra to the ventromedial thalamus and to the superior colliculus of the rat. Brain Res 176:273–283, 1979.
139. Penney JB, Young AB: GABA as the pallidothalamic neurotransmitter: Implications for basal ganglia function. Brain Res 207:195–199, 1981.
140. Houser CR, Vaughn JE, Barber RP, Roberts E: GABA neurons are the major cell type of the nucleus reticularis thalami. Brain Res 200:341–354, 1980.
141. Montero VM, Scott GL: Synaptic terminals in the dorsal lateral geniculate nucleus from neurons of the thalamic reticular nucleus: A light and electron microscope autoradiographic study. Neuroscience 6:2561–2577, 1981.
142. Ohara PT, Sefton AJ, Lieberman AR: Mode of termination of afferents from the thalamic reticular nucleus in the dorsal lateral geniculate nucleus of the rat. Brain Res 197:503–506, 1980.

4

Structural Plasticity of Synaptic Contacts in the Central Nervous System

F.H. Güldner and S.C. Phillips

In this chapter we discuss previous and ongoing work on the normal structure, function and plasticity of the constituents of the synaptic apposition. Presynaptic dense projections have been found to show variability in size between different types of synapses and under different physiological conditions. There are some inconsistencies in the literature with regard to their response to activation or disuse of synapses. This demands further investigations, preferably on defined types of synapses.

The length of synaptic appositions has been found to be highly variable in untreated animals. It appears that either activation or disuse of synapses is less effective in influencing appositional length than is changing the absolute number of synaptic contacts. Neurons appear to maintain a constancy of total synaptic contact area for a given input.

The degree of positive or negative curvature of the apposition appears to be sensitive to various environmental stimuli which influence the activity of synapses. Conflicting results in the literature need to be clarified before definite conclusions can be drawn.

The presence or absence of postsynaptic densities and subjunctional bodies forms the basis of the classification of synapses into Gray type I (similar to asymmetric) and Gray type II (similar to symmetric) varieties. Research has led to the assumption that these structural differences can be equated with excitatory and inhibitory functions respectively. It has been shown that the amount of postsynaptic density material consistently increases after long-term disuse and decreases after long-term activation of synapses. Under these conditions the two classes were found to be interchangeable in optic synapses of the suprachiasmatic nucleus. This has led to the hypotheses that the amount of postsynaptic density material is proportional to the efficacy of excitatory synapses, and some excitatory synapses in the central nervous system can be modified to produce inhibitory contacts and vice versa.

From the Department of Anatomy, Monash University, Clayton, Victoria 3168, Australia.

Current Topics in Research on Synapses, Volume 3, pages 147–169 **© 1986 Alan R. Liss, Inc.**

1 INTRODUCTION

Synapses are recognized as the key sites of communication between neurons in the nervous system. Thus, changes in communication between neurons can be expected to be expressed through morphological and functional changes of the various components of the synapse, particularly the active zone. In this chapter we review various recently performed studies on the active zone, and discuss its contribution to the phenomenon of plasticity in the central nervous system (CNS). Of special interest are the dimensions of the active zone and its paramembranous densities, and the response of these parameters to experimentally induced changes in synaptic activity.

2 PRESYNAPTIC DENSE PROJECTIONS

2.1 Structure, Composition, and Function

The structure and arrangement of presynaptic dense projections (PDP) on the presynaptic membrane have been described in numerous articles [1–6]. PDP are sometimes visible in conventional preparations for electron microscopy (aldehyde/OsO_4 fixation plus uranyl acetate/lead staining of the sections), but they present optimally after impregnation of the tissue with phosphotungstic acid (E-PTA) staining [7,8] and combined bismuth-uranyl-lead (BIUL) staining [2]. PDP appear as triangular, truncated pyramid or polyhedral structures, although they may appear more irregular owing to spikes and actin-like filaments, which connect PDP with a three-dimensional filamentous network in the presynaptic element [4]. The center of the PDP may be more electron-lucent than the periphery [3,4,8], and there is evidence that they are constructed of subunits [3,9–11]. Their chemical constitution is still unclear. On the basis of their staining properties, it has been suggested that the PDP contain proteins rich in basic amino acids [2,12]. There is also evidence for the presence of the proteins stenin [13], tubulin [14], and actin [4].

With the aid of tangential sections it was found that PDP form a triagonal grid (presynaptic vesicular grid) on the presynaptic membrane [2,4,5]. Neighboring PDP are connected to each other by a dense material radiating between their bases. Up to six vesicles can surround each PDP within the grid. While the functional significance of PDP is still unclear, it has been suggested that they guide synaptic vesicles to the presynaptic membrane [1], that dense core vesicles may be involved in the deposition of material on the membrane, or that PDP may be derived from fragments of the shell of coated vesicles [10,15]. It can now also be asked whether PDP provide the framework for presynaptic receptor molecules.

For quantitative analysis it is possible to measure 1) the number of PDP per unit trace length or diameter of synaptic apposition, 2) the base width and height of PDP together with the area of PDP profiles if they are considered as idealized triangles, and 3) the distance between neighboring PDP [3,16].

The size of PDP is variable and is dependent both on the type of preparation and on the synapse under investigation. Their height ranges from 30 to 80 nm and their base width from 35 to 100 nm [2,6,8,17,18]. Their number per apposition can vary considerably; for example, Triller and Korn [6,19] found an average of 2.83 and 2.79 profiles of PDP, respectively, on mean appositional trace lengths of 0.126 and 0.130 μm in two types of inhibitory synapses on the Mauthner cell of the goldfish. Güldner [18] reconstructed 20 synaptic appositions from optic synapses in the suprachiasmatic nucleus of the rat and found that, in medium-sized appositions, the number of PDP was fairly constant at 1 per 0.015 μm^2 appositional area. However, in very large active zones (up to 1 μm in diameter) the number decreased to 1 per 0.03 μm^2, whereas in very small appositions the number is greater at 1 PDP per 0.008 μm^2. The number and size of PDP have been shown to increase during synaptic development [3,20,21], although the size of PDP correlates better with the stage of development than with the number and trace length of the appositions [3].

2.2 Plasticity

Variability in the size and number of PDP in mature synapses suggests that these structures may be important indicators of neural plasticity. Until recently, however, only a few authors had attempted to examine the response of PDP to different types of synaptic activity. While the early studies on PDP should be regarded as nothing more than tentative forays into this area, on account of the inadequate numbers of animals often employed in those quantitative investigations, they nevertheless pointed the way forward for more precise later studies. Jones and Dyson [22] observed a deficit in height and base width of PDP in the cortex of rats undernourished for 7 and for 20 days after birth, in comparison to well-nourished control animals. When feeding *ad libitum* was allowed until maturity, following 35 days of undernourishment, the size of the PDP approached that of control synapses. Quimbi et al. [23] found smaller PDP in the cerebral cortex of rats chronically exposed to halothane during development; these rats also showed learning deficits. Similarly, 18-day-old rats exposed to prolonged repeated hypoxia after birth display shorter PDP in cortical synapses compared with controls [24]. No significant changes in PDP height were found in cortical synapses of adult rats anesthetized with pentobarbital [25], although the number of PDP apparently increased with increasing doses of pentobarbitone [26].

In a specific attempt to correlate morphological and functional parameters Govind and Chiang [27] studied morphological differences between low-output and high-output neuromuscular terminals of the lobster. While these terminals do not have the PDP of central synapses, they are characterized by single dense bars. These workers found that the total PDP surface area was nearly three times higher in high-output synapses (1.14 μm^2) than in low-output contacts (0.41 μm^2). The mean number of PDP per synapse was also higher in high-output (0.73) than in low-output contacts (0.42). However, the mean surface area of PDP was not found to be significantly different between these two types of synapses (0.02 μm^2 in high-output against 0.014 μm^2 in low-output contacts).

Bahar and Güldner (unpublished results) measured the size and number of PDP in optic synapses formed by retinal afferents in the suprachiasmatic nucleus of the rat [18] after constant light or darkness. After 12 h of continuous light influence the PDP were significantly smaller (722.6 μm^2 profile area) than after 12 h of darkness (1,104.1 μm^2). After 2 weeks, 1–2 months, and 8 months exposure to constant light or dark conditions, the PDP appeared larger in "dark rats" than in "light rats," although the difference did not reach statistical significance.There was no difference in the number of PDP per unit trace length of synaptic appositions between the two experimental groups (5.7–5.8/1μm^2 synaptic apposition). In parallel with these results, the PDP in the end bulbs of Held in the ventral cochlear nucleus of rats exposed to either 24 h of silence or repetitive tones in an anechoic chamber [28] were larger after silence (1,418 μm^2, mean profile area) than after sound stimulation (1,342 μm^2). Once again, however, this apparent difference did not reach statistical significance. The numbers of PDP were not significantly different between these two experimental groups.

2.3 Conclusions

Most authors assume that PDP are involved in the release of transmitter, whether this is by drawing vesicles to the active zone and into the presynaptic vesicular grid or by drawing them alongside a presynaptic dense bar. This, in turn, may result in their exerting control over the number of vesicles fusing with the presynaptic membrane during activity [6].

The factors that influence size, shape, or number of PDP remain unclear. It appears that, in mature synapses within the CNS, PDP are smaller in highly active synapses than in comparatively less active contacts [28; Bahar and Güldner, unpublished results]. This may also explain the smaller size of PDP in cortical synapses after prolonged hypoxia, as hypoxia appears to cause increased activity in cortical neurons [29]. It is not clear whether similar conditions apply to cortical neurons after undernourishment [22].

Conversely, in high-output neuromuscular synapses PDP bar-like profiles are larger and more numerous than in low-output synapses [27]. Although the metabolic situation may not be the same in crustacean neuromuscular synapses and neuroneuronal synapses in vertebrates, the different results are puzzling. It needs to be remembered, however, that the dense bars and dense projections have distinct organizational differences and belong to functionally diverse terminals. It may not be wise, therefore, to move automatically from the one to the other. Perhaps the most important principle to emerge from these studies is that the morphology of these presynaptic profiles varies with varying functional demands.

The data gained from developing animals under various experimental conditions are not necessarily of help, since they belong to a large pool of different synaptic types. More studies are needed, therefore, preferably on defined types of synapses, to understand the nature of these important structures. It seems worthwhile considering that PDP may be connected with presynaptic receptors and that a possible up and down regulation of such receptors could be reflected in an increased or decreased size and number of PDP.

3 LENGTH OF SYNAPTIC APPOSITIONS

3.1 Structure and Function

Synaptic appositions (also referred to as active zones, contacts, or junctions) initially appear as short contacts with only a few clear vesicles close to the presynaptic membrane during early ontogenesis. Their length increases with maturation of the contacts and of the paramembranous densities [3]. In a study of synaptic development in the cerebral cortex of unanesthetized rats, Devon and Jones [30] measured a mean contact length of 0.273 μm at 7 days post partum and 0.322 μm at 75 days, with significant fluctuations in between (maximum length 0.337 μm at 10 days, minimum length 0.257 μm). In contrast, Schwarze and Hoheisel [31] found no differences in contact length in developing synapses of the olfactory bulbs on the 1st, 4th, 6th, 9th, and 60th postnatal days. However, there still exists the possibility of fluctuations of contact lengths in the intervals between these experimental days.

An interesting phenomenon is that at least some types of symmetric synapses (similar to Gray's type II [2,3]) tend to have smaller contact sizes than asymmetric ones (similar to Gray's type I). Güldner and Ingham [32,33] measured the mean profile diameter or trace length of apposition in optic and nonoptic synapses of the rat suprachiasmatic nucleus and found that in optic synapses with postsynaptic density thickness of less than 10 nm (clearly symmetric) the mean trace length was 0.19 μm, whereas in synapses with a density thickness of more than 30 nm (clearly asymmetric), the mean trace length was 0.26 μm. In nonoptic synapses symmetric contacts had a mean length of 0.27 μm, whereas asymmetric contacts were significantly longer at 0.32 μm. This confirms the findings of Rutledge [34], who observed a smaller contact length in symmetric synapses compared with asymmetric ones in intact, undercut, and undercut electrically stimulated cortex of the cat. Interesting as these findings are, they provide no indication regarding the significance of the asymmetric–symmetric distribution. They do, however, suggest that these groups represent distinct morphological populations.

3.2 Plasticity

The size of synaptic appositions can be extremely variable even in the same type of synapse. For example, in optic synapses the diameter of three-dimensionally reconstructed contacts ranges from 0.13 to 0.8 μm. The corresponding areas are 0.07–2.5 μm^2 assuming an ideal disk-like shape [18]. By comparison, Govind and Chiang [27] obtained a range from 0.1 to 0.75 μm^2 for neuromuscular synapses of the lobster.

The question remains whether the size of synaptic appositions is determined solely during development, or whether there are additional factors modifying it during adulthood and senescence. It seemed worthwhile, therefore, to examine the influence of high-synaptic transmission activity and also of disuse on this parameter. In our series of studies on the plasticity of optic synapses in the suprachiasmatic nucleus of developing, adult, and senescent rats kept in constant light or dark conditions, the trace lengths of synaptic appositions did not differ significantly between these conditions. Thus the mean trace lengths were 0.238 μm and 0.248 μm, respectively, in rats reared from birth for 4 months in constant light and dark conditions, respectively [35]; 0.266 μm and 0.267 μm, respectively, in adult light and dark rats following 14 days of constant light or darkness, respectively [32], and 0.313 μm and 0.305 μm, respectively, in senescent light and dark rats (Güldner and Phillips, unpublished results). The only difference found was the significantly larger size of appositions in senescent rats compared with young adults (see below for further discussion). No significant differences were found in the mean diameters of the synaptic apposition in end bulbs of Held in the ventral cochlear nuclei after sound stimulation (0.397 μm) and silence (0.419 μm) [28].

In other studies Govind and Chiang [27] measured a mean synaptic surface area of 0.20 μm^2 in low-output neuromuscular synapses (lobster) and 0.18 μm^2 in high-output contacts. The length of synaptic appositions have also been measured in cortical synapses after various experimental conditions in mature and developing animals. There was no significant difference found in the visual cortex and superior colliculus of dark-reared rabbits relative to controls [36,37]. However, Fifkova [38] observed in the upper levels of visually deprived cortex a 7.5% increase in synaptic contact length compared with controls, with deprivation starting on the 14th postnatal day and lasting for 8 weeks. Fifkova [39] also measured axosomatic contacts in visually deprived cortex separately and recorded a decrease of their length following the same treatment. Fisher et al [40] found an 18% increase in lengths of synaptic contacts (lamina II) after prolonged hypoxia during early ontogenesis. This finding is in parallel with decreased cortical thickness (8% less than controls) and a decrease in number of neurons in laminae IV and V. No significant difference was found with respect to this parameter in cortical synapses of undernourished rats at 7, 20, and 112 postnatal days compared with controls [22]. However, in a later study Jones and Dyson [41] found an initial decrease in contact length after 28 days and later an increase after 75 days postnatally in protein-deprived rats. Increasing doses of pentobarbitone have been shown to influence contact length of synapses in the molecular layer of the parietal cortex in rats [26].

Recently, Stewart et al. [42] found an interesting example of lateralization of the medial hyperstriatum ventrale of the chick, where the mean length of synaptic appositions is 12% greater in the right hyperstriatum than in the left one. This difference disappears in chicks after passive avoidance training. The authors did not observe any differences in numbers of synapses per unit volume.

Mollgard et al. [43] observed a significantly smaller contact length of asymmetric synapses in the occipital cortex of rats kept in deprived environments compared with animals kept in enriched environmental conditions. Rutledge [34] found an increase in synaptic contact length in undercut cortex of cat compared with controls, and an even further increase when the undercut cortex was electrically stimulated for 58 days.

One of the most important findings in this regard comes from studies of Hillman and Chen [44,45] on synapses between parallel fibers and Purkinje cells in the cerebellum. The authors observed that after partial experimental elimination of these synapses, the contact area of the remaining synapses increased. This increase was found to be proportional to the number of synapses destroyed. This led the authors to postulate the principle of constancy of contact area. According to this principle, a given neuron tends to maintain the contact area for a given type of afferent after maturation. When synapses of this input disappear later during life, the neuron compensates by increasing the contact area, which presumably brings the input activity back to former levels. This principle may be important when assessing data on synaptic contact lengths, such as those enumerated previously. It also underscores the importance of correlating one parameter with another, such as synaptic number with synaptic size.

3.3 Conclusions

From the available data, it would appear that stimulation or disuse of synapse alone does not cause significant changes in contact size in mature synapses [28,32].

One clear factor would seem to be a change in the number of synapses [45], which in its turn brings about a change in contact size. This principle of compensatory increase in contact area after a loss of synapses could explain the increase in synaptic contact size in the undercut cortex, which has lost a substantial number of afferents [34]. Hillman and Chen's findings [45] also fit in well with the results of Fisher et al. [40], who found increased contact length in cortical synapses after prolonged hypoxia, which is known to cause a loss of neurons and consequently of synapses in the cortex [29]. In senescent rats the contact length of optic synapses in the suprachiasmatic nucleus is increased compared with young adults (Güldner and Phillips, unpublished results). Again, the most simple explanation would be a compensatory response of this parameter to a probable loss of optic synapses at this age (26 months), since numerous degenerating axons were visible in the optic chiasm. Hillman and Chen's principle [45] will have to be tested in other neuronal systems, and further studies are needed to search for other possible factors influencing synaptic contact size in developing and mature nervous systems.

4 CURVATURE OF SYNAPTIC APPOSITION

In a comparative study of synaptic morphology in the spinal cord from pentobarbital-anesthetized and unanesthetized rats, Streit et al. [46] found a significant lifting (increased curvature, convex with respect to the presynaptic element) of the presynaptic membrane in unanesthetized animals. In a series of articles Jones and co-workers studied this phenomenon under various experimental conditions. Thus, Cooke et al. [25] confirmed the results of Streit et al. [46] and found a progressive decrease in the number of such "positively" curved appositions and an increasing number of "negatively" curved synapses (curvature concave with respect to the presynaptic element) with increasing doses of barbiturate [26,30,47,48]. Medosch and Diamond [49] observed more positively curved synapses and fewer negatively curved contacts in the occipital cortex of ovariectomized rats than in sham-operated animals. In the hippocampal (CAI) synapses of rats surviving for up to 60 min after a 10-min-long ischemic insult, von Lubitz and Diemer [50] found an increase in positive curvature compared with controls. Recently, Rees, et al. [28] found a significant reduction in curvature of synaptic appositions in end bulbs of Held in rats exposed to tones compared with rats exposed to silence, although the curvature was still predominantly positive in both experimental conditions.

From the results gained in the end bulbs of Held [28] it would appear that increased synaptic activity causes a flattening of the synaptic apposition. This is in contrast to the interpretation of Streit et al. [46] and Jones and co-workers [26,30,47,48], who found more positively curved appositions together with a more irregular outline of the presynaptic membrane in unanesthetized rats compared with anesthetized animals. These authors thought that the more irregular outline of the presynaptic membrane indicates more fusions of vesicles and, therefore, higher activity in unanesthetized animals. However, it is not yet clear whether pentobarbital dampens the general activity of cortical synapses. Güldner and Wolff [51] and Wolff and Güldner [52] found a swelling of astroglial processes around synapses in the visual cortex of rats after long-term anesthesia with urethane and pentobarbital and after long-term electrical stimulation of the optic nerve. These data could be interpreted in terms of increased activity in the cortex under these experimental conditions. Obviously, more studies are required, preferably on single types of activated and silenced synapses, to clarify these conflicting data.

5 POSTSYNAPTIC SPECIALIZATIONS

5.1 Structure, Composition, and Function

Postsynaptic densities, including subjunctional bodies, have attracted considerable attention since Gray [53] divided CNS synapses into two major classes based upon the presence (type I) or absence (type II) of postsynaptic density material (PDM). General interest increased further following the suggestion that Gray's type I synapses could be excitatory in function and type II synapses inhibitory [54].

Postsynaptic densities were first described by Palay [55] and Gray [53] and may be seen in conventional aldehyde/OsO_4 preparations and poststaining of the thin sections with uranyl acetate and lead salts, after primary OsO_4 fixation, and more selectively after staining with E-PTA and BIUL impregnation (Section 2.1). The focalization of PDM in the developing synapse has been described by Jones and co-workers and by other authors with the aid of E-PTA staining [3,56,57].

In the mature synapse, fixed with conventional methods, PDM appears granular and/or filamentous at high resolution. In a typical asymmetric contact there is a band of PDM directly attached to the postsynaptic membrane, which is highly electron-opaque and variable in thickness (component *a* in Fig. 1, types 1–3). More loosely scattered filamentous material of lesser electron opacity than component *a* (component *b* in Fig. 1, types 1, 2, 4, 5) reaches further into the cytoplasm of the postsynaptic element. As with component *a*, component *b* also appears to be connected

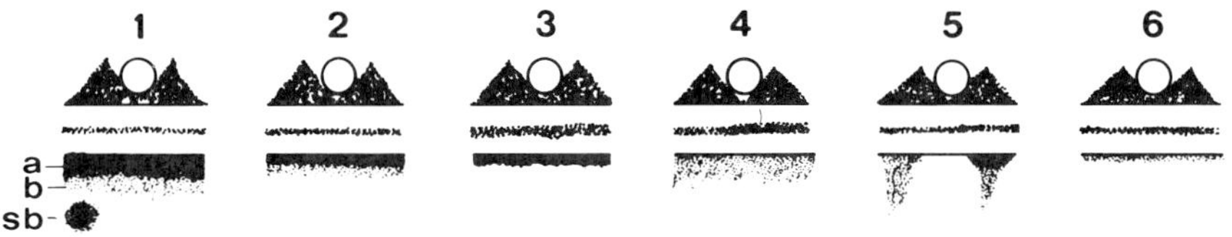

Fig. 1. Schematic drawing of the different types of appositions found in synapses of the rat suprachiasmatic nucleus and other areas of the central nervous system.

to the postsynaptic membrane (Fig. 1, types 4, 5). In a small percentage of synapses only component *a* appears to be present, and its thickness can be less than 20 nm (Fig. 1, type 3). More frequently, synapses with component *b* alone are found. These again have a variable thickness. A relatively small percentage of synapses is characterized by isolated shreds of PDM on a larger apposition. Apart from this feature, this type resembles a symmetric synapse (Fig. 1, type 5); component *a* may or may not be present. Finally, there are synapses that show virtually no PDM; these are symmetric synapses "par excellence."

This classification seems worthwhile, especially since the various PDM forms have not, to our knowledge, been clearly defined or grouped by other workers. A preliminary description of the various PDM forms was given by Güldner and Ingham [33] (see also Rees et al. [28]). Although this classification results from extensive studies on the suprachiasmatic nucleus, ventral cochlear nuclei, and cortex of the rat, it seems to hold true for most other regions in the CNS.

In a number of areas in the vertebrate CNS a variable percentage of asymmetric synapses show *subjunctional bodies* [3,58]. These are distinct, spheroid densities underneath the PDM, with a core of high electron opacity and a less opaque periphery that is connected with component *b* of the PDM. The core and periphery of the subjunctional bodies closely resemble *a* and *b* of the PDM, respectively. Subjunctional bodies appear to be associated only with relatively thick PDM. For instance, in our experience, appositions with thin PDM (20–45 nm) do not show these structures. Serial sectioning of synaptic appositions has revealed that the number of subjunctional bodies is variable. If several of these structures occur in one contact, they lie at an equal distance from the postsynaptic membrane, forming a grid. A percentage of asymmetric synapses in the cerebral cortex and in some other areas show more plaque-like subjunctional densities, similar to the subsynaptic formations described by Taxi [59] in sympathetic ganglia of the frog.

Over recent years the fine structure of PDM has been further elucidated. Matus and others [60,61] have described, with the aid of negative staining on isolated PDM, "a peripheral zone composed of a planar array of spherical subunits with a diameter of 18 nm and one or more islands of fine granular material enclosed by the subunits." Gulley and Reese [62] have shown with the aid of a rapid-freezing and deep-etch technique that PDM in synapses of the anteroventral cochlear nuclei consist of a 20-nm-thick meshwork of 4-nm microfilaments. These fine filaments appear to be connected to particles in the postsynaptic membrane; these are presumably receptors. Granular material fills the interstices of the meshwork of thin filaments. A lattice of thicker microfilaments (9 nm) lies below the meshwork of fine filaments, being intermeshed with the latter and extending up to 100 nm into the cytoplasm. In the same study it was also shown that, following aldehyde fixation, the components of the PDM are clumped together (and represent an artifact). In view of this, it is difficult to compare the results gained with the different histological techniques used. Thus we are unable at this stage to determine whether components *a* and *b* are homologous to the meshwork of fine filaments filled with granules, and the lattice of thicker filaments, respectively. It also needs to be asked whether the spherical subunits observed by Matus et al. [60] are equivalent to the similar-size coarse granules described by Gulley and Reese [62].

In certain types of asymmetric synapses (particularly in the cerebral cortex), the PDM is interrupted by a number of holes or perforations (subsynaptic plate perforations [63,64]). These perforations extend through the synaptic cleft and are always adjacent to the gaps between the PDP. The functional significance of these interruptions is not known, although it has been postulated that they are implicated in the remodeling of synapses in the mature nervous system [65,66].

Much more is known about the chemical composition of PDM than PDP. According to Matus [61], PDM contain a polypeptide of 50,000 mol. wt. (major postsynaptic density protein), actin, tubulin, calmodulin, phosphoprotein I, a high-molecular-weight microtubule protein, and two types of postsynaptic density kinases (one activated by cyclic AMP and the other by calmodulin). Recently, it has been reported that the major postsynaptic density protein is a subunit of a calmodulin-dependent protein kinase [67,68], which phosphorylates itself as well as several other proteins. PDM of at least some synapses contains cyclic 3′,5′-nucleotide phosphodiesterase [69,70], while adenylate cyclase can also occur in the PDM [71]. In all the micrographs shown by these authors phosphodiesterase and adenylate cyclase appear to be associated with PDM of asymmetric synapses. However, it is not yet clear whether these enzymes also occur in symmetric synapses, where their electron-dense reaction product could simulate PDM. Concanavalin A has been shown to bind directly to glycoconjugates under the postsynaptic membrane in symmetric synapses, giving the appearance of a postsynaptic density [72]. It appears, therefore, that an osmophobic material is attached to the postsynaptic membrane of symmetric synapses, and is not stainable in conventional EM preparations. The arrangement of this "ghost density" appears comparable to the PDM in asymmetric synapses.

The functional significance of PDM is still unclear. There is strong suspicion, however, that postsynaptic densities are connected with receptor molecules in the postsynaptic membrane, trapping them in the area of the apposition [61,64]. The regulation of calcium uptake also seems to be an important factor, and in at least some synapses the presence of phosphodiesterase and adenylate cyclase indicates involvement in the second messenger systems. Very recently it has been proposed that changes in synaptic conductance, if maintained for long enough, result in a change in PDM structure [73]. This, in turn, may lead to a change in the pattern of overall CNS conductivity.

The amount of PDM present in synaptic appositions is extremely variable. Colonnier [74] observed a continuum of postsynaptic density thicknesses in cortical synapses. Optic synapses in the rat suprachiasmatic nucleus show an uninterrupted progression of thicknesses from a virtual absence of PDM to the presence of very thick postsynaptic densities with many subjunctional bodies [18]. In this area of the brain, the PDM also displays sexual dimorphism, the mean thickness of the PDM in axospinous synapses being significantly greater in the male rats (29.0 nm) than in females (18.9 nm) [75]. Similar observations have recently been made by Rapisardi and Lipsenthal [76] in synapses of the dorsal lateral geniculate nucleus.

One optic bouton in the rat suprachiasmatic nucleus can make up to five synaptic contacts with different dendritic elements [18]. In each of these contacts, the amount of PDM may vary considerably. One such bouton can even form a clearly symmetric contact with one dendrite, and an asymmetric contact having a thick postsynaptic density with another dendrite (Fig. 2) (see also Güldner [18] and Güldner and Wolff [77]). This could mean that each of these contacts has a different efficacy and that a single optic bouton may induce excitation and inhibition in the different postsynaptic elements [18,77].

The continuity of postsynaptic density thicknesses in synapses creates problems regarding the classical distinction between Gray type I and type

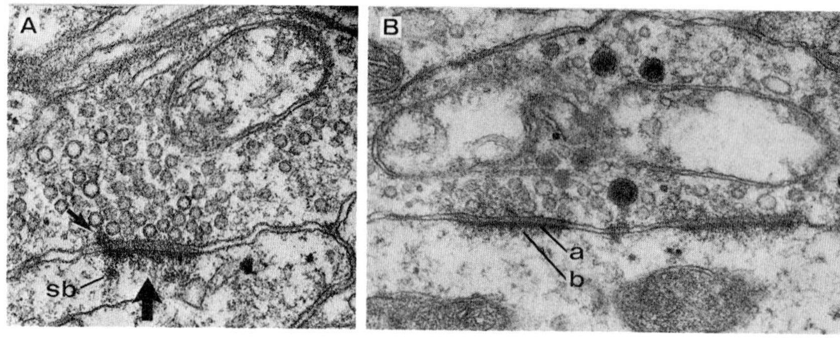

Fig. 2. A. Synapse from the rat suprachiasmatic nucleus with perpendicularly cut apposition showing one presynaptic dense projection (small arrow) and a postsynaptic density (large arrow) with several subjunctional bodies (sb). Note the highly electron-opaque component of the postsynaptic density lying on the membrane and a less opaque component reaching further into the dendritic cytoplasm. B. An asymmetric optic synapse from the rat suprachiasmatic nucleus with perpendicularly cut apposition. Components a and b of the postsynaptic density are clearly distinguishable (See Fig. 1).

II synapses, which are regarded as equivalent to asymmetric and symmetric contacts, respectively. Akert et al. [2] regarded a thickness of 20 nm as a "watershed" between the two classes of synapses: a PDM thinner than 20 nm defining symmetric or Gray type II contacts and a PDM thicker than this being classified as an asymmetric or Gray type I contact. This somewhat arbitrary figure of 20 nm has served well for morphometric studies, especially as the majority of symmetric, inhibitory synapses appear to have PDM thinner than 20 nm and most excitatory contacts having a PDM thicker than 20 nm.

This principle was found in all combined morphological/electrophysiological studies on such synapses [19,54,78–81]. In several other studies excitatory synapses are associated with thick PDM and inhibitory contacts with thinner or virtually no PDM [76,82,83]. The question remains whether there is an absolute boundary somewhere between 10 nm and 30 nm for a postsynaptic density thickness separating inhibitory and excitatory synapses. Alternatively, this arbitrary range of 10–30 nm may constitute a "grey zone" of overlap between some inhibitory contacts with thicker PDM and excitatory synapses with thinner PDM.

In this respect another observation could be important for the distinction of inhibitory and excitatory contacts: the symmetric (inhibitory?) dendrodendritic synapses in the suprachiasmatic nucleus of the rat [84,85] either have no PDM or have material of medium electrondensity (component *b*) rarely exceeding 20 nm in thickness. Highly electron-opaque material (component *a*) has never been found in these synapses. It may be, therefore, that the presence or absence of component *a* is an indicator of excitatory or inhibitory synapses, respectively. If this is the case, a contact with PDM more than 20 nm thick, but consisting only of component *b* (Fig. 1, type 4), may be inhibitory. In the same way, contacts belonging to type 3 and with PDM thinner than 20 nm may be excitatory. This principle appears to hold also for the excitatory contacts of the end bulbs of Held in the cochlear nuclei [28] and it would appear worthwhile to test this possibility in synapses in other parts of the nervous system. Thus, the thickness of the PDM may not be the only criterion upon which to identify a synapse as excitatory or inhibitory.

5.2 Plasticity

The great variability of PDM thickness, even in a single type of synapse under normal conditions [18], raises the question whether this parameter responds to experimental changes in synaptic activity. In order to explore this possibility, optic synapses in the rat suprachiasmatic nucleus were examined in male hooded rats kept in constant light and dark conditions for different periods of time. In a very consistent fashion, the PDM was significantly greater in animals kept in constant darkness (dark rats) than in those kept in constant room light (light rats). This was true for rats reared from birth to 4 months of age under these conditions (postsynaptic density area 0.0059 μm^2 in light rats, 0.074 μm^2 in dark rats, 0.0059 μm^2 in controls [35]), for young adult rats kept in light or darkness for 12 h, 14 days, and 1, 2, and 8 months [32,35; unpublished observations], and for 26-month-old, senescent rats [Güldner and Phillips, unpublished results]. Alongside the increased PDM in dark rats was an increase in the number of subjunctional bodies. The ratio of asymmetric to symmetric optic synapses was also greater in dark rats than in light rats under all experimental conditions. When compared with control animals maintained in a 12 h/12 h light-dark cycle, the dark rats were found to have more asymmetric and less symmetric synapses; the converse is true for the comparison of light rats with controls. As there was never a significant difference in length of apposition or in number of synapses per unit area, we concluded that the changes in PDM occur in existing synapses and are not due to the loss or new formation of optic synapses. In these terms, PDM in dark rats may have been added to existing postsynaptic densities, making them thicker and increasing their profile areas. As a consequence, some symmetric synapses appear to have become asymmetric owing to the addition of PDM. Conversely, in light rats, PDM decreases in existing appositions, producing thinner densities and turning some asymmetric contacts into symmetric ones.

As optic synapses in the suprachiasmatic nucleus show only very thin, unmyelinated axons, they are probably slow-conducting and do not have a high firing rate [18]. This is supported by electrophysiological studies [86]. Statistically significant changes in PDM thickness appear in optic synapses later than 12 h and before 14 days under constant light or dark influence [32]. In view of these results it was of interest to see whether such a change would occur more rapidly in fast-firing synapses. These conditions are met by the end bulbs of Held in the anteroventral cochlear nuclei, which belong to the few easily recognizable types of synapses in the CNS. Thus, these contacts were morphometrically evaluated in young adult male rats exposed to either 24 h of silence or 24 h of repetitive 77-dB tones in a soundproof anechoic chamber [28]. The amount of PDM was found to be significantly increased in contacts of the end bulbs after disuse (silence; mean thickness of PDM 30.44 nm), compared with that in activated synapses (tones; mean thickness 26.04 nm). In activated end bulbs, PDM could become very thin, but the contacts did not completely fulfill the criteria of symmetric synapses. It would be interesting to see whether stimulation for longer than 24 h produces an increase in the number of symmetric appositions in end bulbs.

Increase in the amount of PDM has also been observed in a number of other situations. These include nonoptic synapses in the rat suprachiasmatic nucleus after degeneration of the retinal afferents (bilateral enucleation [33]), synapses of the visual cortex of rabbits after visual training [87], synapses of the hippocampus (CA3) after long-term potentiation [88], and synapses of the sensorimotor cortex of rabbits studied during summation reflex in chronic experiments [89]. In this context, it is important to note that elimination of visual input to the superior colliculi causes an increase in GABAergic terminals with asymmetric contacts [90]. This confirms the data of Lund [91], who found that more boutons with flattened vesicles form asymmetric contacts than do controls. This agrees with our study on the deafferented suprachiasmatic nucleus, where we find a general increase in PDM in the remaining non-optic synapses, whereas a much higher percentage of synapses with pleomorphic vesicles form asymmetric contacts compared with normal conditions [33]. Prolonged continuous administration of GABA (3–7 days) or sodium bromide in the superior cervical ganglion of adult rat induces formation of free postsynaptic densities in neurons [92–94]. This newly formed PDM-like substance does not lie opposite synaptic boutons. It was not determined whether PDM in existing synapses had increased under these experimental conditions.

A decrease in the amount of PDM has been found in cortical synapses of developing rats exposed to prolonged hypoxia [40] and in hippocampal synapses (CAI) after a 10-min-long ischemic insult followed by survival up jto 60 min in length [50].

5.3 Conclusions

The results of these studies suggest that changes in the amount of PDM may indicate changes in efficacy of the synapses concerned. Disuse of synapses, which goes along with an increase in the amount of PDM, appears to induce an increase in efficacy (supersensitivity, hyperexcitability) due to up-regulation of postsynaptic receptors [95]. Such a situation exists in dark rats of all ages, where the optic synapses in the suprachiasmatic nucleus show an increase in amount of PDM compared with normal and light rats. The same happens in end bulbs of Held after auditory disuse [28]. An increase in the number of postsynaptic receptors can also be expected after long-term potentiation, which was found to be accompanied by an increase in PDM in the hippocampus [88]. It would not be unreasonable to assume a potentiation of synapses in the visual cortex after specific training [87] and in the sensorimotor cortex during summation reflex [89]. The results of Wolff and co-workers [92,94] are of special interest in this respect. The long-term influence of GABA on neurons in the superior cervical ganglion causes extreme inhibition, i.e. disuse for several days. The highly supersensitive neurons appear to provide numerous free synaptic sites inviting excitatory innervation. Our hypothesis is, therefore, that an increase in postsynaptic density material generally indicates an increase in efficacy of excitatory synapses and increased excitability of the postsynaptic neuron.

Conversely, continuous stimulation often induces a decrease in efficacy of synapses (desensitization, subsensitivity) due to down-regulation of receptors [96]. This situation occurs in light rats, and in rats kept under continuous noise, where the optic synapses and end bulbs of Held, respectively, show a decrease in the amount of PDM. A decrease in PDM may, therefore, indicate a decrease in efficacy of excitatory synapses and decreased excitability of the postsynaptic neurons. This is supported by Shibata et al. [97], who found that housing rats in continuous light conditions for 10 days suppressed the discharge rate of neurons in the suprachiasmatic nucleus.

The changes in ratio of asymmetric and symmetric optic synapses have been discussed in terms of excitatory synapses turning into inhibitory ones in light rats, and inhibitory synapses turning into excitatory ones in dark rats [32]. This change in quality of synaptic transmission would require a change in type or conformation of postsynaptic receptors in the same neuron. The possibility that one neuron can indeed synthesize different types of receptors for a given transmitter was shown by Alger and Nicholls [98] and Morita and Katayama [99].

It remains to be seen whether neurons postsynaptic to optic afferents are capable of providing excitatory and inhibitory receptors. If this is true, there could be two different types of receptors in the postsynaptic membrane, in varying proportions according to the degree of efficacy. A contact with equal proportions of receptors would then be ineffective, since the inhibitory and excitatory potentials would cancel each other out; this would be a silent synapse. It is tempting to speculate that "goat beards" of PDM in an otherwise symmetric contact (Fig. 1, type 5) may indicate islands of excitatory receptors between areas of inhibitory receptors. Alternatively, if excitatory and inhibitory receptors do not occur together in an active zone, the possibility remains that a desensitized excitatory contact may lose so much PDM that it looks like a symmetric inhibitory synapse but is in fact an ineffective excitatory contact.

It is evident that the morphological, biochemical, and electrophysiological evaluation of the active zone is still in its early stages, although many important advances have been made.

6 ACKNOWLEDGMENTS

The support of the National Health and Medical Research Council of Australia is acknowledged.

7 REFERENCES

1. Gray EG: Electron microscopy of presynaptic organelles of the spinal cord. J Anat (Lond) 97:101–106, 1963.
2. Akert K, Pfenninger K, Sandri C, Moore H: Freeze etching and cytochemistry of vesicles and membrane complexes in synapses of the central nervous system. In Pappas GD, Purpura DP (eds): "Structure and Function of Synapses." New York: Raven, 1972, pp 67–86.
3. Jones DG: "Synapses and Synaptosomes." London: Chapman and Hall, 1975.
4. Le Beux YJ, Willemot J: An ultrastructural study of the microfilaments in rat brain by means of E-PTA staining and heavy meromyosin labeling. II. The synapses. Cell Tissue Res 160:37–68, 1975.
5. Vrensen G, Nunes Cardozo J, Muller L, Van der Want J: The presynaptic grid: A new approach. Brain Res 184:23–40, 1980.

6. Triller A, Korn H: Transmission at a central inhibitory synapse. III. Ultrastructure of physiologically identified and stained terminals. J Neurophysiol 48:708–736, 1982.
7. Bloom FE, Aghajanian GK: Cytochemistry of synapses: A selective staining method for electron microscopy. Science 154:1575–1577, 1966.
8. Jones DG: Some factors affecting the PTA staining of synaptic junctions. Z Zellforsch 143:301–312, 1973.
9. Gray EG: Synaptic fine structure and nuclear, cytoplasmic and extracellular networks. The stereoframework concept. J Neurocytol 4:315–339, 1975.
10. Jones DG, Bradford HF: The relationship between complex vesicles, dense core vesicles and dense projections in cortical synaptosomes. Tissue Cell 3:177–190, 1971.
11. Kadota K, Kadota T: Isolation of coated vesicles, plain synaptic vesicles and flocculent material from a crude synaptosome fraction of guinea pig whole brain. J Cell Biol 58:135–151, 1973.
12. Pfenninger, K: The cytochemistry of synaptic densities. J Ultrastruct Res 34: 103–122, 1971.
13. Berl S, Puszkin S, Nicklas WJ: Actomyosin-like protein in brain. Science 179:441, 1973.
14. Walters BB, Matus AJ: Proteins of the synaptic junction. Biochem Soc Trans 3:109, 1975.
15. Gray EG, Willis RA: On synaptic vesicles, complex vesicles and dense projections. Brain Res 24:149–168, 1970.
16. Jones DG: Quantitative analysis of synaptic morphology. Trends Neurosci 4:15–17, 1981.
17. Güldner FH, Wolff JR: Neurono-glial synaptoid contacts in the median eminence of the rat: Ultrastructure, staining properties and distribution on tanycytes. Brain Res 61:217–234, 1973.
18. Güldner FH: Synapses of optic nerve afferents in the rat suprachiasmatic nucleus. II. Structural variability as revealed by morphometric examination. Cell Tissue Res 194:37–54, 1978.
19. Triller A, Korn H: Morphologically distinct classes of inhibitory synapses arise from the same neurons: Ultrastructural identification from crossed vestibular interneurons intracellularly stained with HRP. J Comp Neurol 203:131–155, 1981.
20. Bloom FE: The formation of synaptic junctions in developing rat brain. In Pappas GD, Purpura DP (eds): "Structure and Function of Synapses." New York: Raven, 1972, pp 101–120.
21. Jones DG, Dittmer MM, Reading LC: Synaptogenesis in guinea pig cerebral cortex: A glutaraldehyde-PTA study. Brain Res 70:245–259, 1974.
22. Jones DG, Dyson SE: Synaptic junctions in undernourished rat brain—An ultrastructural study. Exp Neurol 51:529–535, 1976.
23. Quimbi KL, Aschkenase LJ, Bowman RE, Katz J, Chang LW: Enduring learning deficits and cerebral synaptic malformation from exposure to 10 parts of halothane per million. Science 185:625–627, 1974.
24. Fischer J, Langmeier M, Trojan J: Shortening of presynaptic dense projections produced in the synapses of rat cerebral cortex by prolonged repeated hypoxia in early ontogenesis. Physiol Bohemoslov 29:93–98, 1979.
25. Cooke CT, Nolan TM, Dyson SE, Jones DG: Pentobarbital-induced configurational changes at the synapse. Brain Res 76:330–335, 1974.
26. Jones DG, Devon RM: An ultrastructural study into the effects of pentobarbitate on synaptic organization. Brain Res 147:47–63, 1978.

27. Govind CK, Chiang RG: Correlation between presynaptic dense bodies and transmitter output at lobster neuromuscular terminals by serial section electron microscopy. Brain Res 161:377–388, 1979.
28. Rees S, Güldner FH, Aitkin L: Activity dependent plasticity of postsynaptic density structure in the ventral cochlear nucleus of the rat. Brain Res 325:370–374, 1985.
29. Ribak CE, Bradburne RM, Harris AB: A preferential loss of GABA-ergic, symmetric synapses in epileptic foci: A quantitative ultrastructural analysis of monkey neocortex. J Neurosci 12:1725–1735, 1982.
30. Devon RM, Jones DG: Synaptic parameters in developing rat cerebral cortex: Comparison of anaesthetized and unanaesthetized states. Dev Neurosci 4:351–361, 1981.
31. Schwarze P, Hoheisel G: The postnatal development of synapses at the dendrites of rabbit mitral cells. Acta Anat (Basel) 96:591–599, 1976.
32. Güldner FH, Ingham CA: Plasticity in synaptic appositions of optic nerve afferents under different lighting conditions. Neurosci Lett 14:235–240, 1979.
33. Güldner FH, Ingham CA: Increase in postsynaptic density material in optic target neurons of the rat suprachiasmatic nucleus after bilateral enucleation. Neurosci Lett 17:27–31, 1980.
34. Rutledge LT: The effects of denervation and stimulation upon synaptic ultrastructure. J Comp Neurol 178:117–128, 1978.
35. Güldner FH, Phillips SC: Structural plasticity of developing optic synapses under different lighting conditions. Neurosci Lett 55:225–228, 1985.
36. Vrensen G, de Groot D: The effect of dark rearing and its recovery on synaptic terminals in visual cortex of rabbits. A quantitative electron microscopic study. Brain Res 78:263–278, 1974.
37. Vrensen G, de Groot D: Quantitative aspects of the synaptic organization of the superior colliculus in control and dark-reared rabbits. Brain Res 134:417–428, 1977.
38. Fifkova E: The effect of monocular deprivation on the synaptic contacts of the visual cortex. J Neurobiol 1:285–294, 1970.
39. Fifkova E: Changes of axosomatic synapses in the visual cortex of monocularly deprived rats. J Neurobiol 2:61–71, 1970.
40. Fisher J, Langmeier M, Trojan J: Changes in the length and width of the postsynaptic density, the width of the intersynaptic density and the synaptic cleft in the cerebral cortex synapses of rats exposed to prolonged aerogenic hypoxia during early ontogenesis. Physiol Bohemoslov 29:561–567, 1980.
41. Jones DG, Dyson SE: The influence of protein restriction and changing nutritional status on synaptic development: A quantitative study on rat brain. Brain Res 208:97–111, 1981.
42. Stewart MG, Rose SP, King TS, Gabbot PL, Bourne R: Hemispheric asymmetry of synapses in chick medial hyperstriatum ventricule following passive avoidance training: A stereological investigation. Brain Res 314:261–269, 1984.
43. Mollgard K, Diamond MC, Bennett EL, Rosenzweig MR, Lindner B: Quantitative synaptic changes with differential experience in rat brain. Int J Neurosci 2:113–128, 1971.
44. Hillman DE, Chen S: Plasticity of synaptic size with constancy of total synaptic contact area on Purkinje cells in the cerebellum. Prog Clin Biol Res 59A:229–245, 1981.
45. Hillman DE, Chen S: Reciprocal relationship between size of postsynaptic densities and their number: Constancy in contact area. Brain Res 295:325–343, 1984.

46. Streit P, Akert A, Sandri C, Livingston RB, Moor H: Dynamic ultrastructure of presynaptic membranes at nerve terminals in the spinal cord of rats. Anaesthetized and unanaesthetized preparations compared. Brain Res 48:11–26, 1972.
47. Devon RM, Jones DG: Synaptic terminal parameters in unanaesthetized rat cerebral cortex. Cell Tissue Res 203:189–200, 1979.
48. Jones DG: Synaptic ultrastructure in unanaesthetized and experimentally modified cerebral cortex. "Eleventh International Congress of Anat, Glial and Neuronal Cell Biology." New York: Alan R. Liss, 1981, pp 217–227.
49. Medosch CM, Diamond MC. Rat occipital cortical synapses after ovariectomy. Exp Neurol 75:120–133, 1982.
50. von Lubitz DK, Diemer NH: Cerebral ischemia in the rat: Ultrastructural and morphometric analysis of synapses in stratum radiation of hippocampal CA1 region. Acta Neuropathol 61:52–60, 1983.
51. Güldner FH, Wolff JR: Perisynaptic reactions of astroglia in the visual cortex after optic nerve stimulation. In Creutzfeldt O (ed): "Afferent and Intrinsic Organization of Laminated Structures in the Brain." (Exp Brain Res Suppl 1.) Berlin: Springer, 1976, pp 343–346.
52. Wolff JR, Güldner FH: Perisynaptic astroglial reactions to neuronal activity. In Schoffewiels E (ed): "Dynamic Proportion of Glial Cells." Elmsford, New York: Pergamon, 1978, pp 115–118.
53. Gray EG: Axosomatic and axodendritic synapses of the cerebral cortex: An electron microscopic study. J Anat (Lond) 93:420–433, 1959.
54. Uchizono K: Characteristics of excitatory and inhibitory synapses in the central nervous system of the cat. Nature (Lond) 207:642–643, 1965.
55. Palay SL: The morphology of synapses in the central nervous system. Exp Cell Res 5 (Suppl):275–293, 1958.
56. Dyson SE, Jones DG: The morphological categorization of developing synaptic junctions. Cell Tissue Res 16:363–371, 1976.
57. Rostas JA, Brent VA, Güldner FH: The maturation of postsynaptic densities in chicken forebrain. Neurosci Lett 45:297–304, 1984.
58. Milhaud M, Pappas GD: The fine structure of neurons and synapses of the habenula of the cat with special reference to subjunctional bodies. Brain Res 3:158–173, 1966.
59. Taxi J: Etude de l'ultrastructure des zones synaptiques dans les ganglions sympathiques du Grenouille. C R Acad Sci Paris 252:174–176, 1961.
60. Matus A, Ackermann M, Pehling G: Regularity and differentiation within the structure of brain postsynaptic densities. J Neurocytol 10:889–896, 1981.
61. Matus A: The postsynaptic density. Trends Neurosci 4:51–53, 1981.
62. Gulley RL, Reese TS: Cytoskeletal organization at the postsynaptic complex. J Cell Biol 91:298–302, 1981.
63. Peters H, Kaisermann-Abramof JR: The small pyramidal neuron of the rat cerebral cortex. The synapses upon dendritic spines. Z Zellforsch 100:487–506, 1969.
64. Cohen RS, Siekevitz P: Form of the postsynaptic density. J Cell Biol 78:36–46, 1978.
65. Carlin RK, Siekevitz P: Plasticity in the central nervous system: Do synapses divide? Proc Natl Acad Sci USA 80:3517–3521, 1983.
66. Dyson SE, Jones DG: Synaptic remodelling during development and maturation: Junction differentiation and splitting as a mechanism for modifying connectivity. Develop Brain Res 13:125–137, 1984.

67. Bennett MK, Erondu NE, Kennedy MB: Purification and characterization of a calmodulin-dependent protein kinase that is highly concentrated in brain. J Biol Chem 258:735–744, 1983.
68. Kelly PT, McGuiness TL, Greengard P. Calcium/calmodulin dependent phosphorylations in synaptic junctions. Soc Neurosci Abstr 9:1030, 1983.
69. Florendo NT, Barrnett RJ, Greengard P. Cyclic 3′,5′ nucleotide phosphodiesterase: Cyto-chemical localization in cerebral cortex. Science 173:745–747, 1971.
70. Sugimura K, Mizutani A: Electronmicroscopic cytochemical study of cyclic nucleotide phosphodiesterase in rat brain. Histochemistry 55:97–105, 1978.
71. Panula P, Rechardt L: Ultrastructural demonstration of adenylate cyclase in the rat neostriatum. Neuroscience 4:779–788, 1979.
72. Matus AI, Walters BB: Type 1 and 2 synaptic junctions: Differences in distribution of concanavalin A binding sites and stability of the junctional adhesions. Brain Res 108:249-256, 1976.
73. Siekevitz P: The postsynaptic density: A possible role in long-lasting effects in the central nervous system. Proc Natl Acad Sci USA 82:3494–3498, 1985.
74. Colonnier M: Synaptic patterns on different cell types in the different laminae of the visual cortex. Brain Res 9:268–287, 1968.
75. Güldner FH: Sexual dimorphisms of axo-spine synapses and postsynaptic density material in the suprachiasmatic nucleus of the rat. Neurosci Lett 28:145–150, 1982.
76. Rapisardi SC, Lipsenthal L: Asymmetric and symmetric synaptic junctions in the dorsal lateral geniculate nucleus of cat and monkey. J Comp Neurol 224:415–424, 1984.
77. Güldner FH, Wolff JR: Retinal afferents form Gray Type I and Type II synapses in the suprachiasmatic nucleus (rat). Exp Brain Res 32:83–89, 1978.
78. Reese TS, Shepherd GM: Dendro-dendritic synapses in the central nervous system. In Pappas GD, Purpura DP (eds): "Structure and Function of Synapses." New York: Raven, 1972, pp 121–136.
79. Neale EA, MacDonald RL, Nelson PG: Intracellular horseradish peroxidase injection for correction of light and electron microscopic anatomy with synaptic physiology of cultured mouse spinal cord neurons. Brain Res 152:265–282, 1978.
80. Egger MD, Freeman NCG, Malamed S, Masarachia P, Proshansky E: Electron microscopic observations of terminals of functionally identified afferent fibers in cat spinal cord. Brain Res 207:157–162, 1981.
81. Rastad J: Ultrastructural morphology of axon terminals of an inhibitory spinal neurone in the cat. Brain Res 223:397–401, 1981.
82. Haberly L, Behar M: Structure of the piriform cortex of the Opossum. III. Ultrastructural characterization of synaptic terminals of association and olfactory bulb afferent fibers. J Comp Neurol 219:448-460, 1983.
83. Burry RW, Lasher FJ: Electron microscopic autoradiography of the uptake of [^{3}H] GABA in dispersed cell cultures of rat cerebellum. I. The morphology of the GABA ergic synapse. Brain Res 151:1–17, 1978.
84. Güldner FH, Wolff JR: Dendro-dendritic synapses in the suprachiasmatic nucleus of the rat hypothalamus. J Neurocytol 3:245–250, 1974.
85. Güldner FH: Synaptology of the rat suprachiasmatic nucleus. Cell Tissue Res 165:509–544, 1976.
86. Sawaki Y: Retino-hypothalamic projection: Electrophysiological evidence for the existence in female rats. Brain Res 120:336–341, 1977.

87. Vrensen G, Nunes Cardozo J: Changes in size and shape of synaptic connections after visual training: An ultrastructural approach of synaptic plasticity. Brain Res 218:79–97, 1981.
88. Moshkov DA, Petrovskaia LL: Time dependent changes in the structure of the synapses of hippocampal field CA3 after their potentiation. Tsitologia 25:500–507, 1983.
89. Riabinina MA, Artiukhina NI: Morphofunctional changes in the synapses of the rabbit sensorimotor cortex during the summation reflex. Zh Vyssh Nervn Deiat 30:814–823, 1980.
90. Houser CR, Lee M, Vaughn JE: Immunocytochemical localization of glutamic acid decarboxylase in normal and deafferented superior colliculus: Evidence for reorganization of gamma aminobutyric acid synapses. J Neurosci 3:2030–2042, 1983.
91. Lund RD: Development and plasticity of the brain. New York: Oxford University Press, 1978.
92. Wolff JR, Joo F, Dames W: Plasticity in dendrites shown by continuous GABA administration in superior cervical ganglion of adult rat. Nature 274:72–74.
93. Wolff JR, Joo F, Dames W, Feher O: Induction and maintenance of free postsynaptic membrane thickenings in the adult superior cervical ganglion. J Neurocytol 8:549–563, 1979.
94. Joo F, Dames W, Wolff JR: Effect of prolonged sodium bromide administration on the fine structure of dendrites in the superior cervical ganglion of adult rat. In Cuenod M, Krentzberg W, Bloom FE (eds): "Development and Chemical Specificity of Neurons in Brain Research," Vol 51. Amsterdam: Elsevier/North-Holland, 1980, pp 109-115.
95. Sharpless SK: Isolated and Deafferented neurons: Disuse supersensitivity. In Jasper HH, Ward AA, Pope A (eds): "Basic Mechanisms of the Epilepsian." Boston: Little, Brown, 1972, pp 329–355.
96. Muller L, Pattiselanno A, Vrensen G: The postnatal development of the presynaptic grid in the visual cortex of rabbits and the effect of dark-rearing. Brain Res 205:39–48, 1981.
97. Shibata S, Liou SY, Veki S, Domura Y: Influence of environmental light-dark cycle and enucleation on activity of suprachiasmatic neurons in slice preparations. Brain Res 302:75–81, 1984.
98. Alger BE, Nicholls RA: Pharmacological evidence for two kinds of GABA receptors on rat hippocampal pyramidal cells studied in vitro. J Physiol 328:125–141, 1982.
99. Morita K, Katayama Y: Two types of acetylcholine receptors on the soma of primary afferent neurons. Brain Res 290:348–352, 1984.

Index

U.C.W. ABERYSTWYTH LIBRARY